The Complete Book of

Sleep

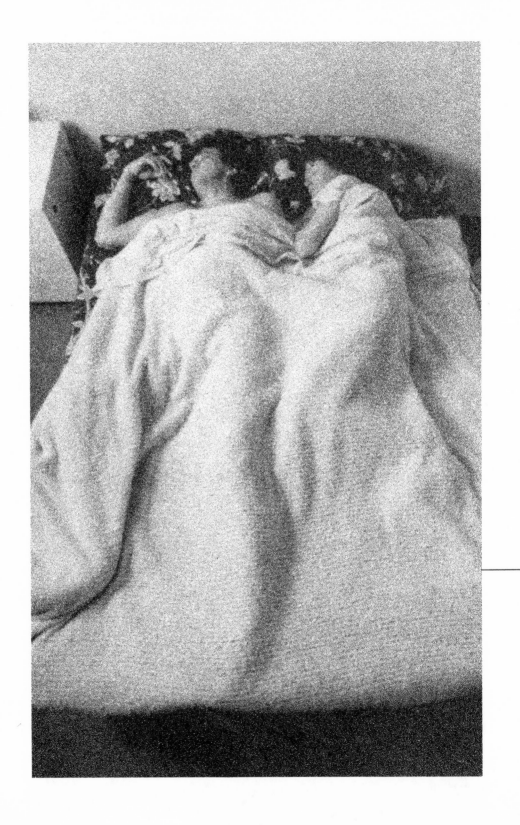

Addison-Wesley Publishing Company

Reading, Massachusetts · Menlo Park, California
London · Amsterdam · Don Mills, Ontario · Sydney

The Complete Book of

Sleep

How Your Nights Affect Your Days

Dianne Hales

Much of the information in Chapter 2 originally appeared in "The Times of Your Life," *Next,*
July/August 1980.

Library of Congress Cataloging in Publication Data

Hales, Dianne R 1950-
   The complete book of sleep.

   Includes index.
   1. Sleep. 2 Sleep disorders.   I. Title.
BF1071.H34   612'.821   80-28150
ISBN 0-201-03845-5
ISBN 0-201-038846-3 (pbk.)

ABCDEFGHIJ–DO–8987654321

For Bob, with love

CONTENTS

PART TWO: SLEEP SENSE

Chapter 6: Sleep Settings: Rocking Your Cradle

*The Way They Slept: The Evolution of the Bedroom •
The Way We Sleep: Bedrooms for All Reasons •
Finding the Bed That's Best for You • How to Buy a Bed •
Tucking Yourself In: Feather Pillows and Rainbow Sheets •
Setting the Temperature for Sleep • Night Noise • Lie Down in Darkness •
Mind Over Mattress*

Chapter 7: Side-by-Side: Sleeping Together

*How the Sexes Sleep • Which is the Weaker Sex by Night? •
How the Sexes Dream •
Sleep and Sexuality: What One Says About the Other •
Sex and Sleep: What One Does for the Other • Two for the Bed •
Coping with Problems in Bed*

Chapter 8: Sleep Styles and Rituals:
Now I Lay Me Down To Sleep

*How Much Sleep Do You Need? • Can You Get By On Less Sleep? •
Nightcaps and Midnight Snacks • Sleep Security •
Sleep Rituals: Whatever Happened to Counting Sheep? •
So What If You Sleep In the Nude? •
Sleep Positions: Night Language of the Body? •
What Your Sleep Time Says About You • Sleeping Off the Job •
Naps: Pajama-Less Sleep • What Not to Do In Bed*

Chapter 9: Techniques to Help You Sleep Better

*Relaxation Techniques •
Cognitive Focusing (Relaxing in the Middle of the Night) •
Self-Management Skills • Stimulus Control • Biofeedback • Hypnosis •
Chronotherapy • Psychological Approaches*

Acknowledgements

This book is a reflection of the work and contributions of many people. I am grateful to the many sleep researchers across the country who provided time, insight and information, particularly to Drs. Rosalind Cartwright, J. Christian Gillian, Ismet Karacan, David Kupfer and Quentin Regestein. I owe a special debt to the staff of the Stanford University Sleep Disorders Center, where I spent many hours learning about the state of the art of sleep research and therapy; I extend my thanks to Drs. Christian Guilleminault and Vincent Zarcone, to Mary Carskadon, Charles Czeisler, Mark Rosekind and Janet Stavosky, and to William Baird, president of the American Narcolepsy Association. Charles Ehret, R. Curt Braeber, Drs. Franz and Julia Halberg, Donald LaSalle, Dr. Charles Stroebel and Dr. Elliott Weitzmann provided help and information on chronobiology and biological rhythms. Eric Hoddes provided an invaluable service by his meticulous reading of the final manuscript. Molly McGinty was an exceptionally helpful researcher, and I am appreciative of the assistance of Grace Tiexera, Beth Edwards and Wolfgang Marleaux.

I also wish to express my appreciation to all the editors I've worked with, on this project and others, at Addison-Wesley. Jane Gillen has been sponsor, supporter and friend. Ann Dilworth helped enormously in organizing and shaping this book. Anne Eldridge orchestrated hundreds of processes to transform the manuscript into a book. I add special thanks to my husband, Dr. Robert Hales, for his enthusiastic and loving encouragement and support and for his many contributions to the book's development.

Introduction

S leep is the stuff of life. We spend a third of our lifetimes asleep, more time than we give to work, to love, or to play. Sleep is the foundation of our health, fitness, and well-being. Yet each night we lay ourselves down to sleep with little awareness of what will happen before we wake. We think of sleep as being passive and uniform, but it actually consists of orderly cycles of complex activity. We think our bodies and brains rest during sleep, but in fact our muscles tense; our pulse, temperature, and blood pressure rise and fall; we are sexually aroused; our senses evoke a world of sights and sounds. We think that in sleep we shed our fears and feelings, but our personalities set our sleep patterns, and our sleep shapes how we feel and act. We accept sleep as commonplace, yet when we cannot sleep, we yearn for it more fiercely than for the rarest treasure. We are able to go without food or water or companionship more easily than without sleep.

Three decades ago the universe of night was unexplored territory, a realm of mystery. In the 1950s, scientists, equipped with sophisticated new monitoring techniques, began unlocking these mysteries. They found that sleep is intimately related to the surges and cycles of hormones and chemicals, that a night of sleep follows an elegant rhythm of sleep stages, that the sleeping brain works in ways distinctly different from, but as intense as those of the conscious mind.

I first reported on the investigations into the frontier of night in 1974. In a crowded basement laboratory of a New York medical center, I learned of the elaborate processes by which scientists study sleep. I watched as volunteers, anointed with dabs of sealing ointment, had tiny electrodes attached to their faces and scalps. With wisps of cotton and dangling wires decorating their heads like tribal ornaments, they crawled into narrow beds to sleep for science's sake. The electrodes on each sleeper sent messages to a "polysomnograph," an elaborate monitoring device that translates a sleeper's brain waves, heartbeats, eye movements, and muscle activity into wavy rhythms scratched out on continuous sheets of paper.

I was as intrigued by those who watched as by those who slept. Who were these students of the night, peering intently not at the sleeper but at those fluttery squiggles? What so fascinated them that they did without sleep themselves in order to observe as others slept? When I looked at a sleep recording, I saw a meaningless and undecipherable hieroglyphic. But the men and women at the monitoring machines had cracked the code. Their excitement was the excitement of an archaeologist or an astronaut, receiving and reading messages from a lost or uncharted world. The revelations from the universe of the night were so new, so unexpected, and so compelling that sleep had become an eye-opening adventure for those who studied it.

I have since written about other researchers and fields of research and about other states of mind and body. But many of the story lines intersected at the same point: sleep. When I wrote about the human heart, I discovered that half of all heart attacks occur at night. When I wrote about mental illness, I found that troubled sleep could be a reflection of a troubled mind. When I wrote about aging, I learned that nothing changes more dramatically in the course of a lifetime than sleep patterns. When I wrote about stress, I saw how sleep enhances our ability to cope with challenging situations. When I wrote about the powers of the mind, I entered the endlessly astounding realm of dreams. I realized that sleep is the crucial factor in any formula for health or fitness, the *sine qua non* of feeling and performing at the peak of our possibilities.

I also recognized that sleep is more than a "story." It is an entirely new field of exploration, as vast and complex as the biomedical sciences that study waking life. I began the research that led to this book because I was fascinated with this new specialty. Since I am among the fortunate sound sleepers of the world, I brought no bias to this work. I asked questions and evaluated answers solely on the basis of one professional need—the need to know and share what is known.

The Complete Book of Sleep is a compilation of what scientists in a wide range of fields now know about sleep. It is based on a year of interviews with researchers, visits to sleep laboratories, seminars and symposia on sleep, surveys of current research, and reports on future directions for investigation.

In traveling around the country to gather data on sleep, I have noted the emergence of sleep as a major new interest in medicine, psychology, biology, and education. This book, written as a bridge from the world of science to the life of the layman, is a synthesis of the most recent investigations of sleep science and of the practical applications of these studies for all who sleep.

The Complete Book of Sleep is as concerned with waking as it is with sleep. It explores sleep in relation to life's rhythms, to growth and aging, to your body's well-being and your mind's equanimity, to sexuality and sex, to creativity, memory, and dreams. If you sleep well at night, this book will make you aware of what happens during sleep and of how your nights affect your days.

If you sleep poorly—night after night, frequently or occasionally—*The Complete Book of Sleep* provides specific, detailed information on the problems that may be keeping you up at night and what can be done to overcome them. One of every two people develops a serious sleep difficulty at some point in life. By understanding your sleep needs and style and by developing your "sleep sense," you can avoid many common sleep problems. By finding out what is behind your problems in falling asleep, staying asleep, or waking too early, or your daytime tiredness, you can learn what to do—and what not to do—to rest more easily.

This book is meant to be the starting point of a quest for better sleep and better understanding of self. However well or poorly you sleep, it will show you how and why your sleep profile is unique, and how your sleep is bound up with heredity, exercise, stress, nutrition, illness, depression, and aging. It examines normal and abnormal, easy and troubled, long and short sleep, weaving sleep into the fabric of conscious existence.

I wrote this book to find out more about sleep as a frontier of human biology. I hope that reading it will enable you to cross this frontier and enrich your days with a fuller understanding of the nights of your life.

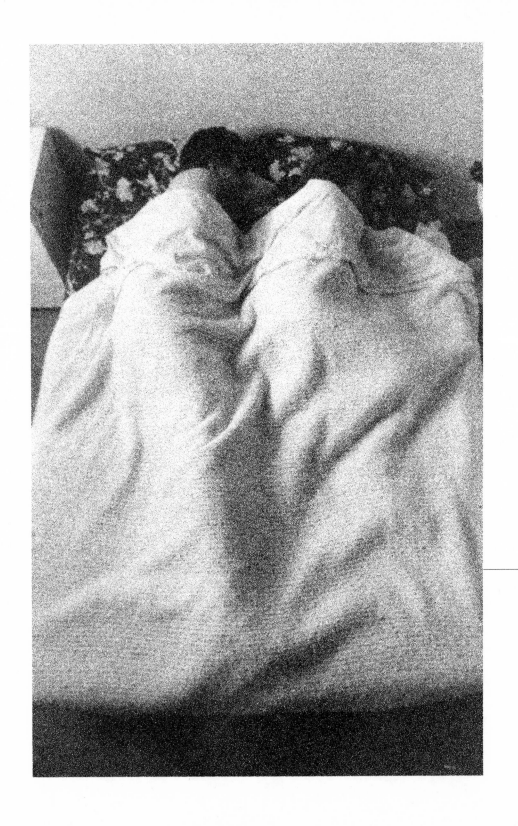

The Facts of Sleep

CHAPTER 1

What is Sleep?

For centuries, sleep has been the basis for myths and mysteries. The people of Fiji thought that the soul went wandering as the body rested, and they were wary of wakening a sleeper so abruptly that the soul might not have time to return to the body. Some ancient cultures thought of sleep as an intermediate state between waking and death. They often feared sleep as a time when a person might slip from night into eternity. Other societies considered sleep a realm of deities and built temples in which to worship the lords of the night.

Is sleep a curse, a spell cast by a malicious god to banish us from the delights of the waking world? Or is it a blessing, nature's way of nurturing the earth's creatures? Do we sleep out of fear, or need, or boredom? Do we all enter the same world when we sleep or do we explore different pathways, some frightening and some entrancing? Why do our brains weave patchworks of familiar and bizarre images as we sleep? Do we dream to entertain ourselves with wondrous stories that defy the logic of daily life? Or are we escaping to another plane of consciousness?

After centuries of sleep, we still have few answers to such questions. The universe of night remains an enigma, so mundane that we willingly sleep right through our journeys into it, yet so complex that it may hold the key to basic processes of life, health, and thought. Shakespeare's poetic vision of sleep has remained remarkably accurate. It is indeed "balm of hurt minds, great nature's second course; chief nourisher in life's feast." Yet sleep does not always—nor merely—knit the body's "raveled sleave of care." It can be a time of peril as well as peace. In the wee hours of early morning, the body becomes colder, less efficient, more vulnerable. Pain tightens its grip. The depressed become

Electrodes attached to this sleeper at the Stanford Sleep Disorders Center monitor eye movements, muscle activity, and brain waves (shown below).

Chris Springmann,
Black Star © 1979.

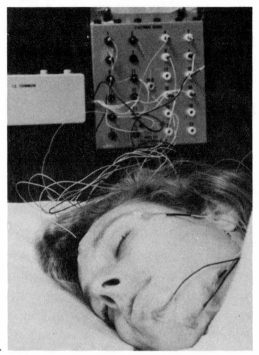

1. EEG (Brain Wave Record) Awake.

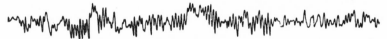

2. EEG Stage 2 Sleep. Brain waves are characterized by sudden bursts of activity.

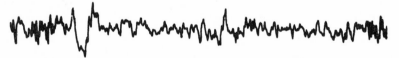

3. EEG Stage 4 Sleep. In this most profound state of unconsciousness, very large brain waves appear in a slow jagged pattern.

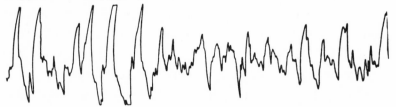

4. EEG REM or "Active" Sleep. Brain waves are pinched and irregular, resembling the patterns of waking more than deep sleep.

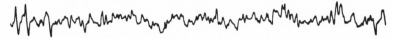

From *A Primer on Sleep and Dreaming* by Rosalind D. Cartwright,
© 1978 by Addison-Wesley Publishing Company, Inc.

desperate. Small children scream in terror at visions they cannot describe. Millions of adults stage nightly battles with the bedclothes, tossing, turning, fidgeting, and fuming in a futile fight for sleep. Sleep difficulties undermine energy and vitality throughout the day; some are so severe that they threaten the lives of people who are perfectly healthy during the day.

Sleep, the common denominator of living things, is a behavior shared by all creatures on earth. Yet it is always highly individual. Your sleep is a sensitive barometer of the state of your life, of your health and happiness, of the nights of your past and the days of your present. The third of your life that you spend asleep is a fundamental part of who you are, how you feel, and what you do.

Portrait of a night

Sleep is a state of mind and body—regular, recurrent, easily reversible, ultimately irresistible. Sleepers look quiet and seem unresponsive to the world around them, but sleep is not a passive state. It is a dynamic process, made up of two types of rest: active and quiet. Active sleep is characterized by movements of the eyeballs beneath closed lids and more intense activity in the brain than during quiet sleep; it is referred to as Rapid Eye Movement or REM sleep. Quiet sleep consists of four distinct stages, all categorized as non-REM or NREM sleep.

Each night you literally turn yourself down for sleep. As you rest, your body begins to slow down, and muscular tension decreases. The brain produces steady, small waves at a rate of nine to twelve cycles per second. In Stage 1 of NREM sleep, your brain waves become smaller and much more pinched, irregular and variable. Mundane thoughts drift through your mind, and pulse and respiration become more even. If awakened from this twilight zone, you may deny having slept. As you enter Stage 2, your brain waves become larger, characterized by occasional sudden bursts of activity. Your eyes become unresponsive to stimuli; if your eyelids were lifted, you would not see. Your bodily functions slow still more, and your eyes may roll slowly back and forth. In Stage 3, your brain waves are about five times the size of those in Stage 1 and much slower (about one cycle per second). In Stage 4, the most profound state of unconsciousness, very large brain waves appear in a slow jagged pattern.

The full journey to the depths of tranquility usually takes more than an hour. Then you begin your ascent, not to consciousness but to active or REM sleep. The muscles of your middle ear begin to vibrate. Your brain waves resemble the patterns of waking more than of deep sleep; they are pinched and irregular. The muscles of your face, limbs, and trunk are slack, but there may be quick bursts of activity in the central nervous system that cause twitches, particularly in the toes and fingers. Your pulse and breathing quicken, and your brain temperature and blood flow increase. Your eyes dart back and forth. Males have erections, whether they are seven months or seven decades old. When sleepers have been awakened from REM sleep in laboratories, 80 percent have reported vivid dreams.

The initial REM period of the night is short, usually only 10 minutes. The 90 to 100-minute REM-NREM cycle is repeated four to five times, with deep NREM Stages 3 and 4 growing shorter and REM periods growing longer during the night. Dreams may occur all through the night, but those recalled from NREM periods tend to be mundane and simple, while REM dreams are usually more dynamic and complex. In an 8-hour night, you will spend 2 hours in REM sleep; in the course of a lifetime, 5 or 6 years are spent in REM sleep and three times that amount in NREM sleep.

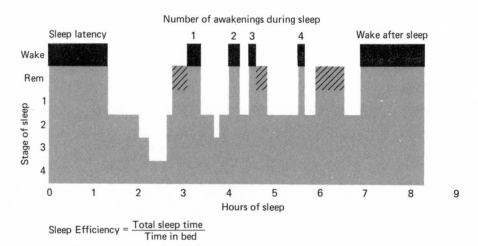

A typical all-night sleep pattern. Courtesy Milton Kramer, M.D., and Thomas Roth, Ph.D.

The Facts of Sleep

As you shift from stage to stage of sleep, your body goes through assorted changes—physical, chemical, hormonal, muscular. Various levels of brain chemicals, including the so-called "sleep juice" serotonin, rise and fall. Body temperature drops to its lowest levels; you breathe less oxygen and burn up fewer calories. In REM, these processes are orchestrated from the brain stem, a region of the brain no larger than your little finger. Your brain, unlike all others in the world, organizes your sleep in a pattern that reflects your sex, age, and health. Your sleep style may be totally different from your bed partner's, but it will be remarkably consistent night after night.

Why do you sleep?

You may assume that each day ends with a night of rest for an obvious reason: the body needs such restoration. All mammals sleep, whether they are great or small, young or old, weak or strong. Where, when, and how much they sleep vary with each species. Sleep needs are not a reflection of the size of an animal's body or the sophistication of its brain. Elephants sleep very little and devote most of their waking hours to gathering food. The small creatures of the night, like the bat and opossum, may sleep more than ten hours a day. Interestingly, the long-sleeping bat has a lifespan of up to eighteen years, while the shrew, about the same size and form but a much shorter sleeper, lives only 2 years. Generally the preyed-upon animals sleep less than the predators of the earth. Cows and sheep sleep in brief snatches; longer naps might separate them from the herd and make them more vulnerable. Gorillas, hunted only by humans, sleep securely for more than sixteen hours a day.

Sleep seems to be nature's way of keeping all creatures out of harm's way. Social scientists have speculated that early humans might never have survived the perils of darkness if sleep hadn't kept them from roaming through the night. The first communities may have formed because of the mutual need to cluster together for safety against dangers in the dark. But perhaps we need no longer fear the night in the neon-lit, round-the-clock bustle of the twentieth century.

Does this mean that sleep has become an anachronism? Not at all, says one eminent sleep researcher, Allan Rechtschaffen, M.D., of the University of

Chicago: "If sleep doesn't serve an absolutely vital function, then it's the biggest mistake the evolutionary process ever made. How could sleep have remained virtually unchanged as a monstrously useless, maladaptive vestige throughout the whole of mammalian evolution while selection has, during the same period of time, been able to achieve all kinds of delicate finely tuned adjustments in the shape of fingers and toes?"

But if there is a timeless need for sleep, what is it? This question remains one of the most perplexing biological riddles. Aristotle thought that we sleep because of a cooling of the vapors of the head. Freud thought sleep was a symbolic journey back to the security of the womb. Pavlov thought of it as a conditioned response. Others have argued that we sleep to repair the ravages of the day, or to purge our brains of extraneous information, or to conserve our energy. Sleep may be maintenance time for our bodies or a sort of dress rehearsal for our brains.

Perhaps none of these explanations is correct. Perhaps they all are, for it may well be that sleep—like waking—has many functions. We may be making an enormous and costly mistake by assuming that our nights are any less significant or complex than our days.

Sleepless nights: the story of Z

There is also an opposite view of sleep: that it is a total waste of time. This was the opinion of a rather eccentric young man—referred to as "Z"—who swore off sleeping at 5:00 A.M. on June 5, 1933. Enlisting the aid of two researchers at the New York State Psychiatric Institute, Z tried to break what he considered a useless and time-consuming habit: his acquired "taste" for sleep. He believed that if he just stayed up long enough he would overcome his need for sleep. To ensure that he would remain awake, the scientists gave him a watchman's clock and key. Every ten minutes he was to turn the key in the lock. After the first night, a friend or relative accompanied him at all times to provide stimulation. Throughout Z's marathon of wakefulness, the researchers carefully monitored his physical functioning, noting changes in heart rate, blood pressure, and other vital signs. They used objective tests to evaluate his mental functioning, reaction time, and muscular contraction strength. Ini-

The Facts of Sleep

tially Z also was given daily typing tests, but after the fourth day they were abandoned; he could no longer focus on the page.

Z steadfastly denied any fatigue of body or of mind. But he began to act like a man who had had one drink too many: irascible, argumentative, disoriented. It became increasingly difficult for him to accept suggestions concerning either his conduct or the course of the experiment. By the third day, Z was reporting dreamlike images and hallucinations. By the fifth day, he seemed in a daze during some of the perception tests. By the tenth day he was incapable of reporting any thoughts.

As days and nights blurred together, Z became convinced that one of the researchers was persecuting him. The delusion grew so strong that the investigators decided to call off the experiment and let Z sleep. Their records showed that, despite precautions, Z had squeezed in about 5 hours of sleep, in snatches from 15 to 70 minutes long. In all, he had gone 231 hours without rest.

Z's record for wakefulness is not unique. In 1959, radio disc jockey Peter Tripp stayed awake without interruption for 200 hours as part of a fund-raising marathon. He appeared unaffected until the final days, when he began imagining that he heard sounds that didn't exist and that unknown enemies were after him. Like Z, he became so suspicious that he refused to cooperate on performance tests.

On the basis of these experiences, researchers theorized that sleep deprivation might lead to a form of mental illness they dubbed "nocturnal psychosis." But these assumptions were challenged in 1964 when a seventeen-year-old San Diego high school student, Randy Gardner, decided to set a record for wakefulness for his school's science fair. Randy stayed awake for eleven days, and while he did grow weary, he did not develop bizarre behavior or hallucinations. He spent the last night of his vigil in the company of a sleep researcher, who testified that he remained rational and pleasant. He held a press conference before going to bed and, after nearly fifteen hours of sleep the first night, resumed normal sleep patterns.

Young, healthy, and motivated, Randy may have been exceptionally prepared to fend off sleep. Yet, like others who try to defy their need to sleep, he ultimately had to succumb. His sleepless nights did not demonstrate how little we need sleep but rather how little we understand and appreciate it. Few of us would ever want to set off on a similar marathon. Quite the contrary: we are quick to register the pangs of a single night's lost sleep. We feel less alert, less enthusiastic, less able to muster our internal resources to accomplish a task. We may function, but with difficulty. Yet sleep loss, though debilitating, is not deadly. There are no records of anyone who died for lack of sleep.

All the sleepy people: where do they all come from?

The fact that sleep loss isn't lethal is small comfort to those who cannot sleep. Just as success is counted sweetest by those who never succeed, sleep is cherished most dearly by those who cannot get the rest they crave. And sleeplessness seems to be part of our human legacy. Even the ancient Egyptians recorded problems of getting to sleep; one of their writings describes the state of being in bed but not sleeping as a living hell.

According to most estimates, one of every three adults—more than 50 million Americans—descends into this hell every night. In the course of a lifetime one of every two persons is likely to have serious problems sleeping. And there may never have been a man or woman on earth who made it through life without a sleepy day or a sleepless night.

Sleep problems are ubiquitous in our society. A survey in Los Angeles found that 33 percent of the respondents had frequent sleep problems, while 42 percent had occasional sleep difficulties. In Florida, 33 to 50 percent of those surveyed reported sleep problems. Studies have shown that sleep complaints increase with age and that women are more likely to report such problems than men. A Gallup poll of 1,550 Americans found that easterners and midwesterners sleep less than southerners and westerners, that more women than men get eight hours of sleep a night, and that high-income earners report more sleep difficulties. Older women may have the highest incidence of sleep problems.

What all these numbers add up to is an epidemic, silent and lonely, that affects millions of weary and bleary-eyed souls. But the actual numbers of the "waking wounded" who stumble through the day may include millions of others who don't connect their daytime daze with their nighttime rest (or lack of rest). Daytime sleepiness may be more prevalent than the common cold. Look around you on the train home; half the passengers may be nodding in their seats. Check the rearview mirror of your car; chances are you'll catch a driver behind you in mid-yawn. With some individuals, daytime sleepiness is a symptom of serious illness. With most of us, it is self-inflicted: we rush to classes, jobs, or chores, starving ourselves of the sleep we need to function at our peak. Without adequate sleep we lose a certain sharpness and zest. Sleepy people score more poorly on performance and I.Q. tests; they are more prone to accidents on the job. The same is true on the highways: in California and Oklahoma, studies have shown that 20 percent of car accidents involve sleepy drivers.

Stanford University researchers have experimented with ways of overcoming daytime tiredness. A daytime nap sometimes provided a boost of energy, but it increased nighttime sleep problems. When college students were allowed to sleep longer at night, they slept less efficiently but were less sleepy in the daytime. When their night sleep was restricted, they slept more efficiently but were more tired during the day. Researcher Mary Carskadon, Ph.D., has postulated that the ideal sleep schedule for the college age group might be a shortened, consolidated period of nighttime sleep plus a daytime siesta.

In other studies, schoolchildren considered to be two to three years behind normal levels quickly progressed and caught up with their peers when allowed to sleep as much as they wished. Older people who slept as long as they chose were less depressed and more energetic. Women who slept more than eight hours a night were rated as less tense and anxious than those who slept less than seven hours. The conclusion of such reports is both eye-opening and unsettling: that many—perhaps even most—of us are less alert, less personable, less competent, and less happy because we are not getting the sleep we need.

The science of sleep: a new frontier

Perhaps the reason that sleep has so often been underestimated is that it has long been misunderstood. Until recently, scientists had no tools to peer within the sleeping body and brain. They put motion detectors under mattresses to monitor body movements in sleep or measured how bright a light or loud a sound had to be to waken a sleeper. Yet it wasn't until the development of sophisticated technology to monitor brain waves (electroencephalogram), eye movement (electrooculogram), and muscle activity (electromyogram) that

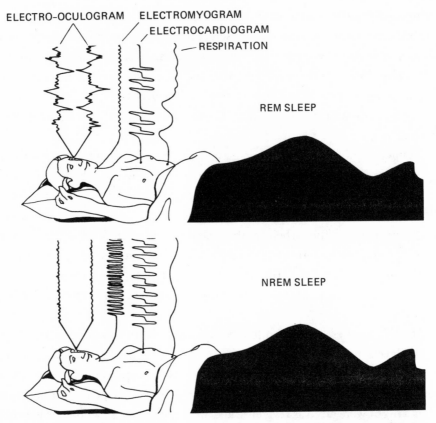

ELECTRO-OCULOGRAM   ELECTROMYOGRAM
ELECTROCARDIOGRAM
RESPIRATION

REM SLEEP

NREM SLEEP

Distinguishing REM and NREM sleep on the basis of all-night sleep recordings. Illustration adapted from THE PSYCHOLOGY OF DREAMING by Robert L. Van De Castle. © 1971 General Learning Corporation. Reproduced by permission of Silver Burdett Company.

researchers gained real insight into what happens during sleep. The biggest breakthrough came in 1954, when scientists at the University of Chicago identified the characteristic pattern of REM sleep and correlated it with dreaming. This discovery marked the birth of a new biomedical discipline.

The field of sleep research has grown rapidly. Two decades ago a department or hospital laboratory devoted only to sleep was almost unheard of. Now there are several dozen sleep centers around the country. In 1976 the Association of Sleep Disorders Centers (ASDC) was formed to "ensure highest quality evaluation and treatment" at these centers and has set up standards for each facility and certification tests for those who work in them. In 1980 the ASDC and the American Association for the Psychophysiological Study of Sleep published its first diagnostic classification, a catalogue of more than 100 distinct disorders, including some that were unknown just a few years ago. But sleep science is still a youngster amid other biomedical fields. "While most medical specialities have emerged over many years, we are trying to collapse a century of clinical evolution into a period of a few months," says William Dement, M.D., director of Stanford's sleep center and a pioneer in the field. As he notes, there are hundreds of thousands of doctors who are trained to care for the disorders of waking life but fewer than fifty who specialize in the myriad problems of sleep. (See Chapter 19 for more information on sleep centers.)

The exploration of the inner space of sleep began about the same time as the exploration of outer space, though from the beginning it has attracted far less attention and support. Yet it already has yielded great dividends for each of us as individuals. Sleep research has helped our understanding of the functioning and organization of the brain, of the natural cycles of our bodies, of mental illness and perceptual problems, of diseases that can claim or cripple lives, of the fundamental changes involved in aging. The universe that sleep research has unlocked may not be as vast as the cosmos, but it is equally intriguing. As scientists listen in on the signals sent during sleep and gather reports from tens of thousands of nights of sleep and dreams, they are developing new insight into the way that the brain, the mind, and the body work as one.

The potential benefits of sleep research are unknown, but its promise is great. Already sleep specialists have helped thousands attain the simple but elusive goal—a good night's sleep. Never in history has there been such effective help for sleep problems, which are some of the oldest of human ailments. And, never before have all of us had such access to the riches and complexities of our night world.

We measure the quality of our night's sleep by the quality of our day's energy. This is what we want from sleep and what we fear we'll lose when we do not sleep. A fuller knowledge of what sleep is and how to sleep better pays off by day as well as night. And this is the best reason for joining in the exploration of the inner world of sleep.

CHAPTER 2

Sunrise, Sunset: The Rhythms of Your Life

To every purpose under heaven there is indeed a season—and a time for every process in every body: a time to be born (4:00 A.M. is the most common hour in humans), a time to die (6:00 A.M. is the fateful hour), as well as times for your heart to speed up and slow down, for your temperature to rise and fall, for your mind to reason and dream.

Rhythm is the essence of your body's time. Like all living creatures, you have rhythm, or more precisely, a distinctive set of rhythms. In the course of a single day, you are constantly and rhythmically changing. There is a pattern to the release of your hormones, the division of your cells, the sensitivity of your taste buds, and the sharpness of your memory. You may be completely unaware of most of these cycles, but one rhythm—that of sleep and waking—is too obvious and too important to be ignored.

All humans respond to the sleep/wake cycle. In frigid Arctic winters and steamy tropical summers, men and women lie down to rest and awaken to work. In the blackness of caves and the quiet of isolation chambers, research volunteers have organized days and weeks into a remarkably uniform rhythm of sleeping and waking. Tuning in to the biological rhythms within and around you can help you understand your own sleep cycles—as well as the clocks and calendars of your entire life.

Going around in cycles

Canute, an ancient Saxon king of Britain, once ordered the tides to cease their daily invasion of his land. Despite all his royal powers, he found himself unable to turn back the ocean's charge against his shores. Centuries later scientists have discovered similarly implacable forces within the human body: rhythmic surges in temperature, blood pressure, respiration, digestion, and other physiological processes. Like Canute, you can rail against the tides within and try to work or sleep or travel in defiance of these internal cycles. Or you can learn to recognize these rhythms and use them to your best advantage.

Different cycles revolve all around you. Each year winter yields to spring, spring to summer, and summer to autumn. Trees and plants bud and bloom and wither. Birds fly south for winter and north for summer, responding to a signal that needs no words or reminders. Many species become fertile only at set times in a yearly cycle, when the sexes begin timeless mating rituals as if on cue.

Even more mysterious are the cycles we cannot observe so readily, particularly those within us. Each month the reproductive system of an adult woman prepares for the possibility of childbearing. Each day your body temperature climbs and falls by a few degrees, and enzymes and hormones are released in orderly sequence.

It wasn't until several decades ago that the complexity of these biological rhythms was recognized and recorded. In the late 1940s, Franz Halberg, M.D., a professor at the University of Minnesota, noticed dramatic differences in his counts of white blood cells in laboratory mice at different times of the day. Monitoring the highs and lows, he charted a daily cycle, which he termed a "circadian" rhythm (from the Latin for "around a day"). Through meticulous daily measurements, Halberg and his colleagues detected and documented rhythms in hundreds of biological processes in mice and men. As a result of this work, chronobiology—the study of rhythmic events in living creatures— emerged as a new way of thinking about life and time.

Why is it that so many cycles are approximately twenty-four hours long? Some scientists believe that at the very dawn of life on earth, the sun, the moon, and the tides embedded this rhythm in the creatures that inhabited the planet. The sun's daily crossing of the sky and descent into darkness was a powerful time cue or "zeitgeber"; the ebbing and flowing of the tides every twenty-five hours in response to the moon's magnetic pull provided another.

These are not the only external factors that affect your internal timing. The temperature of the air, the length of day or night, mealtimes, food, and

The Facts of Sleep

stimulants such as caffeine all influence your body's clock. The strongest time cue for humans seems to be the rhythm of other humans. A baby, born without any strong sense of night and day, sleeps erratically until it begins to mimic its parents' schedule. People of all ages sharing the same house or room or bed invariably influence each other's timing.

In addition to these factors are internal cues, including variations in hormones, levels of sodium and potassium, and changes in brain chemicals. Scientists have shown that the rhythmic changes in body temperature rhythms influence the need for rest periods and the times of peak performance. But the key to biological rhythms, according to some researchers, lies within the brain. In rodents, a small cluster of neurons in a region of the brain called the suprachiasmatic nucleus (SCN) seems to receive time cues from the retina of the eyes and transmit time signals to the animals. However, scientists disagree as to whether humans might have a similar internal time-setter. They have been unable to explain why, when the SCN of animals is removed or destroyed, the natural biological rhythms—altered but recognizable—persist. It may be that the ability to "tell" time is shared by many cells in the brain and body.

Experiments in which volunteers have been isolated from time cues have shown that time sense can be distorted in the absence of external zeitgebers. Most of the research subjects started "free-running" in cycles somewhat longer than the conventional 24-hour rhythm. Some people may naturally follow this longer cycle for waking and resting, particularly those who cannot make use of typical time cues. For example, Stanford University researchers have found that a blind person, unable to respond to light and darkness, lives a daily cycle that averages 24.9 hours and periodically suffers from being out of synch with the world. Shift workers and long-distance travelers may encounter similar difficulties because their cycles are out of harmony with the cycle of life around them.

Such biological rhythms are entirely different from "biorhythms," which have been popularized and publicized. Biorhythms, mathematical formulas for charting mood or energy levels according to one's date of birth, were originated by a German doctor named William Fliess. He believed that everyone is bisexual, expressing so-called male qualities such as strength and courage and female characteristics such as sensitivity and intuition. According to his theory, these character traits surge and ebb in cycles of twenty-three days for male traits and twenty-eight days for female traits. This notion, developed in 1887, might have been ignored if no less a luminary than the great psychiatrist Sigmund Freud had not hailed it as a "great breakthrough in biology." Fliess claimed that he could diagnose neurotic symptoms and sexual abnormalities by examining the nose, correlating his universal cycles with changes in the mucous lining. He treated such disorders with surgery or the nasal application of cocaine. Although Freud became a patient and underwent cocaine treatments twice, he eventually rejected Fliess's work.

However, interest in biorhythms continued, and in the 1930s another cycle—a thirty-three-day rhythm of mental acumen—was added to Fliess's original two cycles. In the 1970s computer firms began offering year-long printouts of an individual's biorhythms, all based on date of birth.

Chronobiologists dismiss these trendy biorhythm calculations as being mathematically incomprehensible and scientifically unsound. Statisticians have tried to determine how vulnerable we really are on the "critical days" when our biorhythms are fluctuating, and in one study, researchers compared reports of more than 13,000 on-the-job accidents and 8,500 air mishaps with the critical days of the workers and pilots. They found absolutely no correlation.

The times of your health

Time is a new dimension for medical thinking, and the serious consideration of changing cycles has upset the classic medical view of health as "homeostasis"—that is, a state of equilibrium within the body. Chronobiology is replacing this freeze-frame picture with images of body and mind in action. In chronobiology, a single measurement at a set time is a tiny piece of a large and complex puzzle. Only by charting changes over time can a biological rhythm be identified and examined.

When we do *what* we do has an enormous impact on our activities. Differences in timing can, for example, be critical in the administration of drugs. The time a medication is taken affects both how effective it is and how long it stays in the body. Aspirin, the most widely used drug in the United States, remains in the body for twenty-two hours if taken at 7:00 A.M. but remains for only seventeen hours if taken at 7:00 P.M.

Some of the exciting research in drug timing involves the powerful medications used against cancer. At the University of Arkansas, Lawrence Scheving, Ph.D., has been using time to target anticancer drugs in hopes of eliminating side-effects on healthy tissue. The drugs, given to mice with various tumors, are administered at times when normal cells and bone marrow are not dividing. "We shield the normal tissue with time," says Dr. Scheving, "the way we shield it with lead during radiation. Our goal is to minimize such side-effects as hair loss and nausea while optimizing our attack on cancer."

The results have been dramatic: In one experiment, 94 percent of the animals given the same medication in the same dose at one time of day were cured, while only 16 percent of those getting the same dose several hours later survived. Timing also protected the animals from the dangers of potent drugs. When a certain drug was given at 2:00 A.M., 96 percent of the animals died of its effects, while only 4 percent succumbed to doses given later in the day.

At the University of Minnesota, physicians have been translating the findings of such animal research into therapy plans for cancer patients. Patients with the same type and extent of cancer, given the same drugs in the same doses, improved more and suffered fewer side effects if chemotherapy began at certain times of the day. In India, physicians have been using temperature rhythms to help plan radiation for patients with cancers of the head and neck. They have found that radiation given at the tumor's peak temperature shrunk the cancers more quickly than the same exposure hours earlier or later.

The body responds to anesthesia in much the same way it does to drugs— that is, in different ways at different times. A patient given a standard dose of anesthetic at certain hours may stir beneath the surgeon's scalpel. Rather than relying on potent but potentially dangerous muscle relaxants, surgeons might be able to schedule operations for times when patients will remain still. Some scientists believe that the success of some procedures, such as organ transplants, may depend not only on the time of day but on the day or week of the operation.

Timing could eventually become part of medicine's therapeutic strategy. Drugs might be given for treatment of certain symptoms, such as pain, precisely at the times of greatest flare-up. Insulin doses might be varied throughout the day to correspond to a diabetic's fluctuating blood sugar levels, and antiseizure medications could be administered according to the rhythms of an epileptic's attacks. It is possible that hospitals might even arrange their schedules to provide services according to their patients' optimal time for treatment.

A greater recognition of biological rhythms also could lead to advances in preventive health care. The detection of changes in the regular rhythms of blood pressure could lead to earlier diagnosis of hypertension (high blood pressure), the silent killer of thousands in the industrialized nations of the West. As chronobiologists point out, people who schedule their annual physical exams for early morning might always have normal readings. If they were tested again in late afternoon, their blood pressure might have risen to ominously high levels. Eventually those at high risk of developing hypertension might wear portable monitors around the clock for several days a year so physicians could study their blood pressure rhythms.

A similar strategy might lead to earlier detection of some cancers. At the University of Glasgow in Scotland, Hugh Simpson has theorized that even a tiny cancer of the breast might disrupt monthly temperature rhythms. He designed a brassiere with a built-in electronic device to monitor temperature, and in experimental trials, the device recorded abnormal breast temperature rhythms in women who showed no other signs of cancer. A year later these women were examined again, and this time conventional medical tests showed that a remarkably high percentage of them had developed tumors.

Yearly or "circa-annual" rhythms may prove even more important than daily or monthly cycles in detecting and treating illness. In monitoring these fluctuations over decades, Franz Halberg, the father of chronobiology, has detected slight but significant changes in the amplitude and frequency of certain cycles (how much and how often a function varies). He hypothesizes that these variations may be the cause of the secondary diseases of aging or that they may reflect the primary process of aging. "If we could intervene in some way—perhaps with drugs—to keep our rhythms identical to what they were in youth and maturity," he says, "we might be able to stop or slow down natural aging."

Chronogeneticists, who look beyond one's life rhythms to hereditary sources, have a similar theory. At the Gregor Mendel Institute of the University of Rome, researchers have found parallel timetables for disease and death in identical twins. It may be that our genes carry more than codes for brown eyes or red hair; they may be biological calendars for the timing of illness and the duration of life. According to the geneticists, genes are like candles of different lengths on a birthday cake—some are certain to burn out faster than others. What if we could anticipate which ones will flicker first? Could we keep them burning to preserve health and extend life? Scientists in the United States believe that genes do not necessarily determine destiny. In one experiment, researchers bred mice that were prone to high blood pressure and premature death by stroke. By adjusting the animals' biological rhythms in various ways, they were able to delay the expected time for onset of hypertension.

Such intriguing studies may encourage the hopeful Ponce de Leóns among us, forever questing for a fountain of youth. At the very least, they are revealing a great deal about the nature and needs of aging. One expert in biological rhythms, Charles Ehret, Ph.D., of the Argonne National Laboratory in Illinois, believes that one underlying problem of the aged may be mistiming of basic rhythms, what he calls "circadian dis-synchronization." Physicians examining older patients have observed that various physiological processes no longer work in harmony and certain organs are most active while others are at rest, as if they had missed a critical cue.

Mind time, mood rhythms

Within the cycle of day and night are other, briefer rhythms. While your watch divides the day into twelve 60-minute hours, your body and brain mark time by longer hours. Every 90 minutes there are regular fluctuations in your energy levels and attention span that affect how well you learn new information, remember old data, and respond to sudden stress.

The human "biological hour" grows longer with age. Babies shift from rest to activity roughly every 60 minutes; as they mature, this hour gradually stretches out. Your 90-minute hour is longer than that of small creatures (a rat's biological hour is only 10 to 13 minutes long) and shorter than that of larger animals (an elephant lives by 120-minute hours). You may not be aware of feeling different every 90 minutes, but scientists have documented rhythmic fluctuations in appetite, in the urge for a cigarette or drink, in drowsiness, and even in the tendency to daydream. Some scientists have theorized that early humans needed to have regular peaks in attention and motor skills to facilitate food-gathering and exploration of their surroundings. The subsequent decline in activity might have favored assimilation of food and consolidation of information.

However, not all of your powers of mind and body peak in harmony. Canadian psychologists conducted day-long tests of verbal and spatial skills, administering tests to eight volunteers at fifteen-minute intervals. The subjects regularly scored their best marks approximately every ninety minutes, but when they did best on the spatial tests, their verbal scores were at their lowest.

It may be that each of us performs best not only at ninety-minute intervals but during a certain part of the day. Biological rhythms may also affect learning as well as performance. Chronobiologist Donald LaSalle, Ph.D., director of the Talcott Mountain Science Center in Connecticut, studied variations in students' ability to learn and do well in class. For many students, morning was not the best time to learn; many reached their intellectual peak much later in the day.

There seems to be a correlation between brain function and body temperature. In most people, body temperature is lowest between the hours of 2:00 and 4:00 A.M. and highest from 2:00 to 4:00 P.M. Those whose temperatures peak earlier in the day have been characterized as "larks" because they rise bright and cheery in the morning. "Night owls" require more time not only to wake up but to warm up; their temperatures may not peak until late afternoon or early evening. "Woe be to the child who is an owl in an early morning class in a difficult subject taught by a teacher who's also an owl," says LaSalle. "He has three strikes against him." The mistiming of American education may be one reason why "Johnny"—or rather millions of Johnnys and Janes—can't read. We may be wasting young minds, not by lack of effort but by wasting the effort in trying to teach young minds that are too sleepy to learn. If primary and secondary schools made their timetable for teaching more flexible, students, trained to recognize their mind rhythms, would be able to choose morning or afternoon classes in key subjects. At the very least, teachers might rotate subjects every day so that each topic is taught at different hours during the week. Tests, particularly the standard examinations so crucial for college admission, could be given at different times of the day, rather than only early in the morning.

Mood rhythms as well as mind rhythms may be helpful in the recognition and treatment of emotional problems. Some psychological disorders are characterized by fluctuations in mood. A manic depressive, for example, rises to frenetic highs of nonstop activity and then crashes to despairing lows. At the Institute of Living in Hartford, Connecticut, psychiatrist Charles Stroebel, M.D., has been practicing "chronopsychophysiology" since 1965. Twice a day the staff nurses summarize the physical and mental characteristics of the psychiatric inpatients and feed the information into computers. The patterns that have emerged have enabled Stroebel to anticipate sudden mood swings and to time therapy—including drugs, behavioral techniques, and psychotherapy—according to critical periods. More than 2,000 patients at a behavioral medicine clinic at the Institute of Living are using another technique for understanding the clockworks of body and mind: a standardized diary with questions on body functions, feelings, and life events. The daily tear-out sheets are processed by computer every two weeks. "This is an effective therapeutic tool," says Stroebel, "because it increases awareness of self-destructive things—like sleepless nights or heavy drinking or increased isolation—that patients may have denied or failed to recognize."

Such self-insight could be a possible weapon against the most common cog in our clockworks: stress. All of us can recall times when the same minor incident—such as a flat tire or a spilled glass of milk—triggered rage on one day and only irritation on another day. Far more serious and perplexing are times of unrelieved stress, such as periods of mourning or drastic life change. Such crises can disrupt our normal rhythms, even shortening our biological hour from ninety to sixty minutes. Recognizing these changes and adjusting to them can be critical in rebuilding our sense of confidence and competence.

Disturbed mind rhythms, most apparent at night, may also be clues to mental illness. Normally the cycle from NREM to REM sleep and back again is 90 to 100 minutes long. The first REM period generally begins an hour after we fall asleep and is relatively brief. However, the rhythm and timing of REM and NREM periods is markedly different in patients with certain types of depression. They start dreaming quite early in the night, often in less than 40 minutes. They also tend to awaken early in the morning and are unable to return to sleep. Some psychiatrists believe that this abnormal sleep pattern may be a biological marker of a mental illness, a way of accurately diagnosing and determining the severity of depression. Studies of the unusual sleep of the depressed also have led to some experimental approaches to treating depression, including a night of sleep deprivation and other attempts to manipulate the patient's mental clock (see chapter 5, "The Sleeping Brain").

The correlation between body temperature and performance may also lead to new insight into specific sleep disorders. In experiments at Stanford University and Montefiore Medical Center in New York City, Charles Czeisler, Ph.D., found that the circadian rhythm of body temperature determines how long we sleep. Body temperature was more strongly associated with how long volunteers slept than how long they had been awake before going to bed. It also affected when they started REM sleep and how much time they spent in REM throughout the night.

Temperature cycles may explain why some "night owls" find it impossible to fall asleep when they go to bed at the hours most people do. After hours of thrashing and turning, they usually fall asleep at 3:00 or 4:00 A.M. Czeisler, who began to experience this problem when he was commuting frequently from the East Coast to the West Coast and back again, theorized that his body clock was out of synch with his environment. To reset it, he gradually moved his bedtime around the clock, tinkering with his internal rhythms until they were in phase with the schedule he wanted to keep. This approach, dubbed "chronotherapy," has since become an effective therapy for patients with delayed sleep-onset insomnia (see page 179).

Circadian disorders might also be the underlying problem in other sleep disturbances. Some people's internal clocks may be permanently set on a cycle that is longer or shorter than twenty-four hours. Or daily habits, such as drug use and long naps, or emotional upsets, may throw off the body's timing mechanism. Resetting this delicate self-timer is critical, since living out of harmony with the rest of the world may lead to problems of mind and body during night and day.

Changing shifts and shifting time zones

Over 13.5 million Americans—18 percent of the nation's work force—work full or part-time on evening and night shifts and know how difficult it is to try to "beat the clock." Millions of others inflict on themselves an ailment unique to the twentieth century: jet lag. These night workers and distance travelers share a common interest and problem—sleeping.

Shift workers regularly get less sleep than others—an average of only 5.6 hours (compared to 7.5 hours) every 24 hours. They rarely sleep more than 7 hours at a stretch. Usually they wake up after 4 or 5 hours of sleep, feeling tired and edgy. Even after years on a night shift, many workers never really adjust to their schedule.

Theoretically it should be possible to make a 180° shift in the hours of waking and sleep. However, this is far easier on paper than on the job or in bed. Work performance and efficiency are lower among night workers. Researchers found that meter-readers in a Swedish gas works factory made more errors at night, steel workers had slower reaction times, and phone operators took longer to answer incoming calls. Charles Ehret, an expert on biological rhythms, describes night as the time of your lowest efficiency and energy. You are prone to make trivial mistakes: thinking right and turning left, pushing the up button when you want to go down, misreading maps and instructions. The miscalculations that led to the most serious mishap in the history of United States nuclear energy at Three Mile Island were made at 4:00 A.M. by workers who had been changing shifts every week.

The problem with such a schedule is that workers never get a chance to settle into a rhythm. Usually the body needs three or four weeks to shift to a totally new time frame. Many workers try to live two lives—as night owls during the workweek and as day people on weekends. The stress of this effort shows up in frequent reports of gastrointestinal problems in shift workers as well as marital upsets and emotional disruptions.

The long-term effects of living and working around the clock may be even more serious. One sleep researcher who has studied this problem, Wilse Webb, Ph.D., of the University of Florida, Gainesville, writes: "We are homogenizing the 24 hours and arbitrarily turning people off and on around timeless machines, continuous processes and insatiable output demands. As a consequence, the biological nature of man is being unnaturally bent, and all of the accrued adaptive systems, such as families and group membership, are affected. [These disruptions] will continue into perpetuity since there is no likelihood that man's nature will change to accommodate man's failure to recognize himself as his own worst enemy."

Anyone who attempts to travel around the world in eighty hours can testify to the strain that Space Age technology can put on our Stone Age bodies. For most of us, jet lag is a temporary, episodic problem, but it's an occupational hazard for flight crews. Pilots and stewardesses regularly complain of an array of problems, including headaches, burning eyes, digestive disorders, loss of appetite, shortness of breath, menstrual irregularities, and chronic sleep problems. Among the folklore of flying is the belief that crews who fly east-west routes age more quickly than those who fly from north to south.

Scientists have provided reasons to take such notions seriously. At the University of Minnesota, two groups of mice were observed on a schedule of twelve hours of darkness and twelve hours of light. At the age of fifty-eight weeks, the light-dark cycle was inverted for one group, as it might be if they had been flown halfway around the world. Their lifespan was 6 percent shorter than that of the mice who stayed on a steady schedule.

Pilots' well-being is particularly critical, not only to themselves but to their passengers. Newspapers regularly report "near-miss" stories about pilots asleep at the controls. In one incident, three crew members on an all-night flight from New York to Los Angeles flew right over the city and out over the Pacific Ocean. The air traffic controllers, frantically trying to reach them by radio, finally managed to awaken one of the crew after the plane had traveled 100 miles west of Los Angeles. Fortunately they had enough fuel to make a quick turnabout. Some serious air crashes in recent years have been traced to mistakes made by crews who had been flying and sleeping on irregular and demanding schedules.

Sleepiness is not the only symptom of jet lag, however; the digestive system, hormones, and basic metabolism are all thrown out of rhythm. The organ that may be affected most—and that may need the most time to recover—is the brain. United States Army studies of the effects of transatlantic flights on troops airlifted to Europe for NATO maneuvers found that soldiers required up to seven days to recover their ability to think clearly and logically. Their reaction times weren't necessarily slower but they were erratic. The brain fatigue associated with travel may actually be more hazardous than physical weariness. A better understanding of the dangers of living or flying "out of rhythm" may lead to different schedules for flight crews and manipulation of external time cues to lessen the impact of moving too far too fast. Current experiments suggest that tinkering with such pace-setters as diet, caffeine, and rest schedules may help travelers' brains and bodies readjust more quickly when they reach their final destination. (See page 237 for further discussion of shift work and jet lag.)

Health and harmony

Timing is emerging as an important fundamental principle in medicine, biology, and science, as it has been in philosophy, literature, the fine arts, and the performing arts. Chronobiologist Franz Halberg foresees a day when all people will be taught a basic "chronobiologic literacy" that would enable them to use their own rhythms as tools for self-knowledge. The skills of "rhythmometry" are simple enough for schoolchildren to master: in Minnesota and Connecticut, students of all ages have been taught to monitor their body time. Six times a day they check their oral temperature, heart rate, respiratory flow, grip strength, mental quickness, sense of time, energy, and mood. Such self-scrutiny has resulted in the detection of a number of cases of juvenile hypertension as well as a better understanding of daily cycles. One twelve-year-old, trained in self-monitoring, informed her surgeon father that she was coming down with something. He doubled-checked her 98°F temperature and scoffed at her diagnosis. "But Daddy," she argued, "my normal waking-up temperature is 97°." Hours later she was proved right: by late afternoon an inflammation of her lymph glands pushed her temperature up several more degrees.

An understanding of chronobiology can reveal the complexity of your body and your relationship to a rhythmic universe. The sense and science of rhythms ultimately may offer you an opportunity to rewrite *Ecclesiastes* in your own time frame: to recognize within yourself the time to reap and the time to sow, the time to get and the time to lose, the time to embrace and the time to be far from embracing. Chronobiology offers a key to harmony within, an order and peace that may be a prerequisite to harmony without.

CHAPTER 3

Nightlife:
What Goes on When the Lights Go Down

W e all live two lives. In one we are conscious in mind and active in body. We work, play, love, talk, eat, travel, read, and busy ourselves with dozens of tasks. Our other life is spent behind closed lids. "Those who are awake have one world in common," Heraclitus wrote centuries ago. "Those who are asleep retire every one to a private world of his own." Your sleep realm may be as much of a mystery to you as it is to others. You may assume that it is a state of utter stillness, as if your sleeping body were a car parked for the night—engine off, headlights dimmed, motionless, and quiet. It is anything but.

Sleep is a time of intense physical activity, even though you use less oxygen, burn up fewer calories, and rarely speak or rise from your bed. Much of your body's activity during sleep is invisible to an observer. The muscles of your middle ear contract. The flow of your gastric juices changes. The chemicals essential for the basic processes of life pulse silently through your body; some key hormones reach their peak concentrations in your blood as you sleep. A man's penis rises rhythmically; a woman shows subtler signs of sexual stimulation.

You sleep differently when you are young and when you are old, when you sleep alone or with someone, when you are well and when you are ill. The quality of your sleep, however, does more than reflect your waking life; it actually foreshadows the quality of your days. Sleep is the foundation of your well-being, your energy, and your appearance. The way you sleep is, quite simply, the way you are.

Sleepy genes: your sleep legacy

According to one tale popular among sleep researchers, a young sleepwalker woke up suddenly on one of his nocturnal sojourns to find himself in the family living room. To his dismay, he was not alone: several of his relatives were also strolling through the room, all sound asleep.

Sleep patterns—and problems—do indeed run in families. Biologists, in careful studies of laboratory mice, found that heredity played a substantial role in how long and deeply they slept, as well as in the rhythms of their activity and rest periods. In humans, the best evidence for heredity's influence comes from the study of twins, both those derived from a single egg (monozygotic) and those conceived from separate eggs (dizygotic). Whether awake or asleep, the brain waves of monozygotic, or identical, twins are essentially alike—even when they have been raised apart. Both identical and fraternal twins show no significant differences in sleep onset (the time needed to fall asleep), sleep duration, or time spent in the various stages of sleep. Identical twins also follow the same rhythm in fluctuating between NREM and REM sleep.

Differences in genes may explain why one person thrives on only four hours of sleep while another needs eight just to stay awake until noon. But you may inherit more than a familial sleep style; the children of parents with sleep problems are much more likely to develop the same disorder. When both parents reported problems in falling asleep in a study published in 1976, so did 48 percent of their offspring. When only one parent had the problem, 29 percent of the children did. By comparison, only 18 percent of children whose parents had no problems in falling asleep stayed awake long after the lights went out.

The correlations with other sleep disturbances are even more striking. In a study of thirty-four navy recruits who were observed walking in their sleep during training, researchers found that 56 percent had sleepwalking relatives. None of sixty other sailors, who stayed in bed through the night, had any relatives who walked in their sleep. There also was a familial link between sleepwalking and bed-wetting: 62 percent of the adult sleepwalkers reported a current or past problem of bed-wetting, and 38 percent had family members with similar problems.

Narcolepsy, a disabling disorder of the sleep-control mechanisms characterized by daytime "sleep attacks," loss of muscle tone, and disturbed night-time sleep, afflicts only .05 to .1 percent of all Americans; however, 2 percent of the first-degree relatives of narcoleptics are afflicted. An estimated 12 to 33 percent of narcoleptics come from families with a history of this ailment. In three generations of one family, eight relatives developed narcolepsy.

The nights of our lives

Before birth we may spend our time in the darkness of the womb in a state similar to sleep. Medical scientists have suggested that sleep, particularly active sleep, is the natural state of the fetus. A baby born prematurely will spend up to twenty hours of the day asleep; 80 percent of this time will be in a REM-like state in which its eyes are closed but its face or limb muscles move. Newborn infants sleep up to sixteen hours a day (though some sleep much less) and continue to spend half of that time in active sleep.

Nothing changes more in the course of a lifetime than sleep patterns. From infancy, your total sleep time decreases by more than half; your REM periods dwindle to less than a quarter of your night's sleep. Even though you don't "learn" to sleep, you do learn how to time your sleep. In the first weeks of life, babies sleep and awaken erratically around the clock. Gradually they begin to consolidate their sleep into periods that are several hours long.

The sleep problems of infants, like their sleep patterns, are different from those of adults, but they are no less serious (see page 253 for more information on the sleep problems of infancy). The most common cause of death in babies less than a year old—Sudden Infant Death Syndrome—may be a form of sleep apnea, a breathing impairment that occurs episodically in sleep. This tragic and mysterious disorder may be caused by immaturities in the child's nervous system. The peril subsides after the baby's first birthday.

Children spend more time than adults in NREM Stages 3 and 4—those of deepest sleep. This time, during which growth hormone is secreted, seems to be critical for healthy development, yet it is also when specific sleep problems—sleepwalking, sleep-talking, bed-wetting, and night terrors—

occur. While these disturbances are fairly common, they are not a threat to a child's health, and most children outgrow them. Despite the problems they experience during the night—including imagined dangers as well as real sleep problems—children are awesomely energetic by day. A group of eight-year-olds or ten-year-olds may seem to be in perpetual motion, and unlike their often exhausted parents, they find it almost impossible to nap during the day.

Daytime sleepiness may be one of the earliest signs that a child is reaching the age of puberty. At a summer sleep camp for children at Stanford University, researchers found that the children who became the most weary during the day were those on the verge of the hormonal changes of puberty. Many teenagers need more sleep than adults or their younger siblings and may sleep ten hours a night *and* nap in the afternoon. Some biologists theorize that teenagers' need for so much sleep is part of nature's preparation for the years of childbearing. Teenage girls seem especially prone to uncommon sleepiness shortly before their menstrual periods.

By age eighteen the sleep patterns of adulthood begin to emerge. But the next few years can be even more tiring than the teens, not because of physical changes but for social reasons. Off on their own in a world of unexplored options, young adults may stay up half the night and sleep in the next day. Even if they follow regular schedules during the week at college or work, they may shatter any such routine on weekends. The not uncommon experimentation with alcohol and drugs during this time can compound the problem.

As men and women in their twenties settle down, their nights take on a regular pattern. They spend about 5 percent of the night in Stage 1 sleep; 50 percent in Stage 2; only 8 percent in the deep slumber of Stages 3 and 4; and the rest in REM. By their thirties, men begin to sleep fewer hours and somewhat less deeply; by age sixty, they have very brief Stage 4 periods. Women sleep deeply longer; they begin spending less time in Stage 4 sleep in their fifties. For both sexes, the onset of middle age may mark the beginning of restless nights of light sleep and more awakenings. By age sixty-five, 40 percent of men and women complain of sleep problems, often only to be assured by doctors that light, fragmented sleep is "normal" for people their age.

It is common, yes. But is it normal? Some sleep researchers have speculated that the poor sleep patterns of the elderly may be symptoms of serious diseases rather than signs of aging. If the need for sleep decreases with age, daytime

The Facts of Sleep

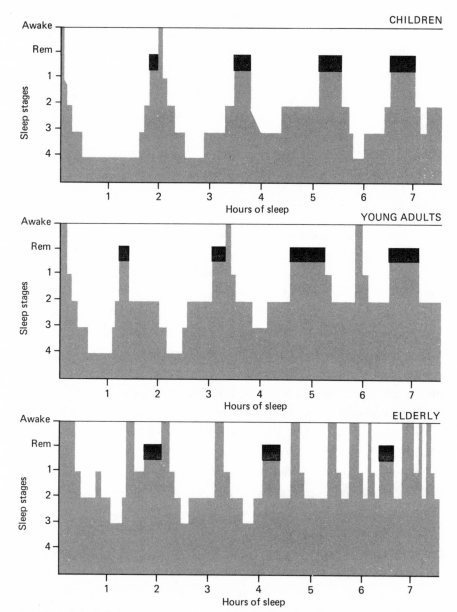

An idealized night's sleep in children, normal young adults, and the elderly.
Adapted from Kales, A: Sleep and dreams. Recent research on clinical aspects.
Annals of Internal Medicine 68: 1081, May 1968.

Nightlife: What Goes on When the Lights Go Down

alertness should remain the same. If the need for sleep remains the same but isn't met, daytime alertness, concentration, and memory may deteriorate—as they often do in the elderly. In a study of sleep patterns in the healthy aged, Patricia Prinz, M.D., of the University of Washington, found that those with the best intellectual functioning spent the most time in REM, while those with lower REM levels showed signs of cognitive decline. Which comes first, the decrease in REM or the decline in brain function? Prinz's conclusion was that "sleep changes may be a factor influencing the process of neurobiological aging and senescence." Other studies have suggested that older people who sleep as well as they did in middle age remain sounder in body as well as in mind.

In sickness and in health

Sleep problems may be both the cause and effect of serious physical and mental woes. Too little sleep—as well as too much—can be hazardous to health and to life. According to a large-scale study of health habits by the American Cancer Society, adults who sleep much less or much more than average are more likely to die prematurely. The researchers found that 99 percent of those adults who slept seven to nine hours each night were alive and well six years later. The mortality rate among men who slept less than four hours a night was 2.8 times higher; among women it was 1.5 times greater. At the other extreme, men and women who slept more than ten hours a night had a death rate 1.8 times above the normal sleepers. Those who took sleeping pills regularly were 1.5 times more likely to die than those who did not.

What happens during sleep may be a life-or-death affair. Stanford University researchers discovered that during REM sleep the hearts of otherwise healthy persons can stop beating. This pattern of nocturnal asystole (no heartbeat) may be responsible for sudden cardiac deaths in normal young adults. At Stanford, four patients twenty-eight to thirty-three years old had nocturnal pauses in their heart rates ominous enough to require permanent implantation of cardiac pacemakers. Daytime tests had failed to reveal any heart disease, and only recurrent chest pain in the night brought these men to the Stanford sleep center for evaluation.

Another potentially lethal disorder of sleep is apnea, a condition of episodic breathing stoppages that last for 20 to 130 seconds and occur as often as 500 times in a single night. One of every four otherwise healthy men over the age of sixty-five may develop apnea; among sleep clinic patients over sixty-five, the incidence is close to 50 percent. The constant struggle to breathe rouses the sleeper, although usually not to the point of awakening, and so disrupts his sleep patterns that he may be irresistibly sleepy the next day. The chronic interference with normal breathing and circulation may also increase the risk of heart disease. (See pages 192 and 227 for descriptions of the various types of apnea.)

Some sleep researchers talk of an "internal medicine of sleep" for diseases that appear only in the night. These ailments can be as debilitating and life-threatening as any which occur during waking hours. "It is possible for individuals to be entirely normal awake and deathly ill asleep," says William Dement, M.D., of Stanford. He foresees a day when patients might undergo a "sleep physical" as routinely as any other regular health exam. Measuring cerebral blood flow, heart function, breathing, nervous system activity, metabolic processes, and other functions during sleep might provide valuable clues to serious diseases and prompt quick action to counter them. At the National Institute of Aging, researchers have monitored the nightly sleep patterns of men and women of ages forty to seventy in order to relate specific sleep abnormalities to the development of certain diseases. Such a "prediction profile" could serve as a valuable tool of preventive medicine and as a method of forecasting and possibly forestalling death.

It certainly seems more than coincidental that half of all heart attacks and more than half of all strokes occur during the night. Patients afflicted by many other diseases also feel worse during the night (see page 244): epileptics have more seizures, asthmatics wheeze more, chronic lung disease patients gasp for oxygen, eczema and psoriasis patients itch. REM sleep triggers more cases of retinal hemorrhage—bleeding in the eye—in diabetics than any daytime activities.

The bodies of the healthy and the ill may function quite differently in sleep. Ulcer patients may produce more gastric acid at night, and some researchers believe that stressful dreams increase acid levels. Another digestive disorder that plagues many sleepers is gastrointestinal reflux, a regurgitation of the stomach contents into the esophagus. Patients with kidney disease, inluding those undergoing dialysis, frequently complain of sleep disturbance. Generally they get less deep NREM sleep and less total sleep, and their REM-NREM cycles are not well organized. It may be that severe kidney disease causes irreversible changes in the brain's functioning, including the way in which it controls sleep.

Sometimes a sleep problem is a symptom of unsuspected disease. Excessive daytime sleepiness can be a clue to the existence of a tumor in the region of the brain known as the hypothalamus. Epilepsy may be diagnosed by evaluating a patient's EEG after a night of normal sleep and after a night without sleep. Sleep problems can accompany the onset of multiple sclerosis and endocrine disorders.

In other cases, the treatment of illness leads to sleep problems. Hospitals are notoriously difficult to sleep in, and several studies have documented the disruption and fragmentation of sleep, particularly in the Intensive Care Unit. Deep sleep may disappear and REM declines. The sleep loss of these desperately ill patients may contribute to the mental disorientation that psychiatrists refer to as "ICU psychosis." Many hospital patients tend to sleep shallowly for ten to twelve hours a day in fragments so brief that they never awaken feeling rested. Deep sleep and REM may disappear for long periods in convalescence, and this lack may impair the natural healing process.

Pain may be the most common disrupter of sleep, whether it comes in the form of arthritic aches or postsurgical discomfort. Pain seems to become more acute at night, possibly because there are fewer distractions from it or because of circadian changes in the brain chemicals that regulate pain sensitivity. While sleep is the patient's only way to retreat from pain, the use of sleep-inducing medications is only a temporary solution. The pills lose their effectiveness within days, and 20 percent of those who become addicted to sleeping pills get hooked while hospitalized.

Sleeping under the influence

What you eat, drink, inhale, smoke, or swallow by day affects how you sleep by night. Such ubiquitous stimulants as nicotine and caffeine can disrupt sleep (see pages 182 and 184). The pills you take for assorted ailments of mind and body can affect your ability to fall asleep and your progression through the stages of sleep. But of all the substances associated with sleep, none is more commonly used—or abused—than alcohol.

About 10 percent of all the prople who drink are alcoholics. Many trace their drinking problems back to when they first tried to drink themselves to sleep. Enough alcohol, drunk quickly enough, can indeed shorten the time it takes to lose consciousness. However, there is a difference between stupor and sleep, and excessive amounts of alcohol invariably create more sleep problems than they solve—or dissolve. Heavy drinking takes its toll in the second half of the night: the sleeper awakens and soon wishes to be anything but conscious. With a pounding heart, a dry mouth, aching muscles, and a throbbing head, every part of the drinker's body feels miserable.

Alcohol shatters the regular rhythms of sleep. Drinkers sleep less, often in brief fragments of rest spread over a longer period of time. REM is suppressed, causing more wakefulness in the morning hours. The hangover that begins at night persists through the day. To get to sleep on the following night, drinkers have to consume more alcohol more quickly, a need that grows as they continue to drink their way out of wakefulness.

When regular drinkers "hop on the wagon," their greatest test comes at night. During withdrawal, the percentage of REM rebounds, and their nights are filled with bizarre, terrifying nightmares. They have problems falling asleep and staying asleep. These sleep disturbances may persist for as long as six months after withdrawal. The most severe alcoholics may end their withdrawal agonies with a "terminal sleep," deep and refreshing. Those with delirium tremens, after days of relentless activity and wakefulness, fall into this sleep and awaken from it lucid and quiet.

Alcoholics may not sleep normally for weeks or months after they stop drinking. Sober ex-drinkers may continue to have gross abnormalities in their NREM-REM cycles and may spend less time than usual in deep NREM sleep. As measured by the EEG, they may suffer irreversible brain changes, although no one knows the long-term consequences of these disruptions.

The effects of other recreational drugs, like marijuana, are similar to alcohol. Some pot-smokers puff their way to sleep, smoking two or three joints as quickly as possible to induce sleep. The following morning they awaken early, after a night of shallow, broken sleep, feeling tired and depressed. Heavy marijuana smokers show gradual deterioration in their ability to function through the day, including lack of motivation and defects in short-term and long-term memory.

Alcohol and marijuana become more dangerous—sometimes deadly—when combined with other drugs, including those regularly prescribed for sleep problems. Since many sleep drugs remain in the body for long periods of time and show cumulative effects, even a few drinks can have unexpectedly dramatic results. The best advice for those in search of sleep is to steer clear of any and all drugs. Even a few late-evening nightcaps can disrupt the normal rhythms of sleep.

Sleep fitness

Perhaps no one appreciates sleep more than those who must perform at peak physical levels during the day. For athletes in every sport, sleep is as important as training. Chris Evert described sleep as her "number-one priority" during competition play. In a survey of the New York Yankees, most of the players said they preferred to get at least nine hours of sleep each night during the season. The purpose of curfew for athletes, coaches explain, is to make sure they get the sleep they need.

Athletes are particularly worried about daytime tiredness because fatigue is a hazard; they might become careless and misuse their bodies, increasing the likelihood of injuries. Coaches try to avoid workouts that lead to exhaustion to avoid the errors and injuries that might jeopardize a career. Sports medicine experts believe that ignoring the need for sleep and rest may lead to athletic "burn-out." Good nutrition alone is not sufficient for the body to recuperate from the physical and psychological stress of competitive sports. Athletes who do not get enough sleep may lose weight, energy, motivation, and interest in their sport. Yet many athletes who "go stale" increase their daytime activity rather than their nighttime rest. They extend their workouts and drive themselves harder. Or they try to distract themselves in a hectic flurry of off-the-field activities. And the problem gets worse.

Why do athletes need more sleep than their fans in the bleachers? Fatigue results from too little body sugar, too much lactic acid, too much heat, too few electrolytes, too little glycogen, and too many metabolic wastes, their coaches say. Only in sleep can these imbalances be righted again.

Sleep is also crucial for another essential factor in athletic performance and competition: timing. As studies with sleep-deprived subjects have shown, too little sleep not only slows down reaction times but also makes them erratic. A sleepy person may react in average time on one test and three times more slowly on the next. Other effects of sleep deprivation—an inability to concentrate, sensitivity to pain, blurred vision, distorted spatial perception—can also keep an athlete or his team out of the running.

Amateur runners, tennis players, and swimmers would also do well to get the rest they need. At the very least, they should watch out for the warning signals of being overexercised and underrested: a feeling of lightheadedness on rising, a racing pulse, early morning or multiple awakenings through the night, feeling so listless that workouts are a chore rather than a pleasure. These signs indicate that it is time to head for the bedroom, not the gym.

Night and day

In recent years good health has become a preoccupation of many people and an obsession of some. You may count calories, jog, eat organic foods, work out with weights, learn to take your own readings of pulse and blood pressure. Yet your quest for fitness by day can be undermined by poor sleep at night. Sleep loss can shatter your timing, your resilience, your zest for life, and your sense of well-being. Good sleep is the basis for feeling good.

Your nights and your days, your sleep and your self, are intricately intertwined. You don't stop being male or female, young or old, healthy or ill, fit or flabby, drunk or sober when you crawl into bed. Your sleep is a reflection of who you are and what you do when you are awake, just as your waking hours reveal either the glow of good sleep or the strain of a bad night.

Your nightlife is too important for you to ignore. By becoming more aware of your sleep, you will begin to understand the many ways in which your days and nights affect each other. Your sleep can send you messages about the state of your body—whether you are becoming ill, pushing yourself too hard, or drinking or eating too much too late. Your sleep can be both a mirror of the days past and a foundation for better days ahead.

CHAPTER 4

The Dreaming Mind

Dreams are a window into the mind. They may be our most elaborate, distinctive, revealing, and flamboyant creations, and they have fascinated us since ancient times. The Egyptians built temples for dreaming. The oracles of Greece pondered cryptic dreams for messages from the gods. Modern psychiatry has viewed dreams as "the royal road to unconscious." Dreams allow us to glimpse beyond that which we are and know in daily life; they hint of other dimensions of space and time. However, the process of dreaming is a mundane one, regular and rhythmic, not unlike digestion. Just as the body breaks down food, the mind processes images from the past and present.

What do your dreams really mean? Are they mirrors of your days, tunnels into recesses of the unconscious, or no more than the chance results of biochemical changes in the brain? No one knows the complete answer yet, but dream researchers are learning more and more about the reasons why we tell ourselves stories as we sleep and how these tales reflect and relate to waking life.

Creative dreaming

In the jungles of Malaysia live a primitive people called the Senoi whose entire society is based on their dreams. The children are taught to report their dreams each morning and to control the frightening ones. They are told to incorporate the messages of dreams into their waking lives. Like all children, Senoi children describe dreams of frightening animals or monsters. By the time they are adolescents they no longer have nightmares, and they consistently derive creative insight from their dreams. How do they make this transition?

Fathers, mothers, and grandparents instruct the children in ways to alter their dreams. Their first rule is always to confront and conquer danger in dreams. Next the dreamer should move toward pleasurable experiences. The third step is to give the dream a positive outcome that yields a creative product.

The Senoi carry these principles into waking life. A dreamer who has been aggressive or uncooperative to someone in a dream makes friendly gestures toward that person while awake. If attacked by someone, the dreamer tells the person of this aggression so they can renew their friendship during the day. Patricia Garfield, Ph.D., a psychologist who studied the Senoi, believes that their translation of dream messages into waking behavior may help solidify their peaceful, cooperative culture. Violence of any sort is rare in their society. The Senoi share each other's food and land and lives. Perhaps their most striking characteristic, she reports, is "their extraordinary psychological adjustment. Neuroses and psychoses as we know them are reported to be nonexistent among the Senoi."

American dream researchers have tried to apply the Senoi dream techniques in our far more advanced and far more troubled culture. The initial studies failed to show that it is possible—or impossible—to control a dream. In other experiments, dreamers tried to improve themselves: before they fell asleep, they repeated a statement about the characteristic they most wanted to change. Frequently, they would display this negative quality in their dreams—with considerable self-enjoyment. It may be that our usual waking moral values are not applied in dreams. If anything, we may be more honest about the gratification we get from faults during dreams.

But even if you can't reshape your character, you can use dreams to develop self-insight. Dream researcher Rosalind Cartwright, Ph.D., studied forty-eight patients who were identified as potential early dropouts from insight-oriented psychotherapy and offered a two-week pretreatment program. Two-thirds of the patients were monitored in the sleep lab. Half of those monitored in the lab were awakened during REM periods and were given access to their vivid dreams; the other half were awakened as often but only from NREM sleep. The "controls" were the patients who went directly into treatment without the sleep monitoring. All of those who slept in the sleep center discussed their nightly dreams. After ten treatment hours, Cartwright looked for correlations between focusing on dreams and successful psychotherapy. She found that those who recalled and discussed their dreams stayed in therapy at a significantly higher rate and used the hours more productively.

Some people use their dreams to help them reach very specific goals. Marathon swimmer Diana Nyad, preparing to swim from Cuba to Florida, repeatedly dreamed of moving slowly through the water toward the white sand of the coast. Golf pro Jack Nicklaus recalls a bad slump early in his career. One night he had a dream in which he was using a different kind of swing and hitting the ball well. The next day, changing his grip to duplicate the dream, he started shooting in the 60s after a string of weeks of scoring in the upper 70s. The German chemist Friedrich Kekule worked for years to discover the structure of benzene. In a dream he saw six snakes biting each other's tails in a circle. This hexagon, he later realized, was the molecular structure for benzene.

But scientists have had little success in studying problem-solving in dreams. Stanford researchers gave 500 student volunteers a problem to study fifteen minutes before bedtime. In the morning each reported any dreams recalled from the night and suggested possible solutions. In 1,148 attempts, only 7 students came up with a correct solution in a dream.

The key to creative dreaming may be the individual's concern and involvement with the problem. The more daytime effort that has gone into solving a problem, the more likely it is for a solution to turn up in the night. In many instances, the person has exhausted nearly all possible solutions during the waking hours. Perplexed yet committed to finding a solution, the person lies down to sleep, and dreams may reveal what was hidden to the overworked waking mind. It could be that all of us are presented with possible solutions to our problems in our dreams, but we either ignore or forget them. "Perhaps only the most perceptive dreamers possess the ability to recognize a solution that is presented in a disguised or symbolic fashion," says sleep researcher Dr. William Dement, who cites a personal example of a dream that helped him tackle a troublesome problem: his heavy smoking of cigarettes.

One night, at a time when he was smoking up to two packs a day, Dement dreamed that he looked at an ominous shadow in his chest X ray and realized that his right lung was infiltrated with cancer. A colleague confirmed that the cancer had metastasized (spread) and that he would not live much longer. "I will never forget the surprise, joy and exquisite relief of waking up," he says. "I felt reborn." He also quit smoking immediately.

Reflections of the day

Dreaming reflects living. At night you dream about the things and people that are important to you during the day. If you are preoccupied with issues of ambition or intimacy, you'll mull them over by night as well as by day. And your processing of such matters will be as mundane in a dream as it is in your waking thoughts—or so some dream researchers contend. Dreams are generally no more scintillating than waking life, they say. "There are peak experiences, isolated snatches of life which truly capture intense romantic exciting feelings," says Milton Kramer, M.D., of the University of Cincinnati. "Let's say you remember five dreams a week. That's five out of 35. If you let me select five experiences out of 35 in my life, I'd have the most fascinating life that's ever been lived." He believes that we tend to forget our dull dreams and remember the more exciting or bizarre ones, including our bad dreams.

Dreams seem to be negative by nature. Yet in one study, in which spontaneously occurring bad dreams were compared with imaginary nightmares, the invented dreams were much more dramatic. Perhaps our secret fears tend to be rather banal. Or perhaps our notion of what a nightmare should be has been overly influenced by Grade-B Hollywood movies.

Yet some dreams can be productions not unlike Hollywood extravaganzas. Cartwright has described a definite sequence to some nightly dreams, organized like a made-for-television, five-part serial. After the characters and plot are introduced in the opening segment, there are flashbacks and flash-forwards and restatements of the central theme, all culminating in an extravagant final dream (the one we're most likely to recall). There is even a dream equivalent of television reruns—recurring dreams that are played again and again within the sleeping brain. Such repetitive dreams are not uncommon, and the unpleasant ones outweigh the pleasant ones two to one. In examining the dreams of 167 women between the ages of eighteen and fifty-five, Cartwright found that 65 percent experienced the same dream at least three times. Of the 220 dreams described, 159 were unpleasant. In another study of male and female students, 64 percent of the women and 54.5 percent of the men had recurring dreams; again, the majority of the dreams were unpleasant. The themes of the bad dreams included being attacked or threatened with injury or death, experiencing a supernatural encounter, being a failure in some social role, and helplessly watching violence. "The dreamer returns again and again to the same scene, like a record stuck in a groove," says Cartwright.

There does seem to be a "typical" dream, which consists of two characters plus the dreamer, occurs indoors, is more passive than active, and is more hostile than friendly. Generally more strange males than females appear, and they are the focus for most of the hostility in the dream.

This dream scenario changes with age. The dreams of childhood are quite simple, no more sophisticated nor frightening than the day-to-day world of the young dreamer. When children under ten have bad dreams, they usually see themselves as being threatened by some evil force, like a monster. It isn't until adolescence that dreamers experience acute embarassment in social situations.

Dreams and symptoms

Dreams may be as intimately related to the body as they are to the mind. In a study at the University of Connecticut, a psychologist found that alcoholics who dreamed about drinking craved alcohol more the following day. The noncravers—the alcoholics who could control their desire for a drink—reported dreams of gratification during the preceding night.

At McGill University in Canada, Harold Levitan, M.D., has investigated the content of patients' dreams in relation to their physical symptoms. The dream patterns of those with specific illnesses were striking and "as characteristic of each diagnosis as were the phenomena of waking life." Among patients with rheumatoid arthritis, a crippling illness in which the body attacks its own tissue, Levitan found four repetitive dream themes: acts of extreme cruelty; becoming the victim of extreme violence; incest, usually with a parent; and dreams in which other people expressed the dreamer's repressed feelings. In many of these dreams, the person's ego seemed too weak to defend the self, so the dreamer became the victim. Levitan believes that the trauma of such dreams—perhaps greater than any stress of waking life because the unconscious has no defensive mechanisms to protect itself—may trigger significant changes in the dreamer's body, changes that could cause or exacerbate certain illnesses. Since the body is unable to distinguish between actual stress and the simulated stress of dreams, it responds with identical chemical changes that could drastically affect the person's health and well-being. For example, one patient dreamed that he carried a violin case onto a stage, removed a machine gun from it, and proceeded to blow his brains out. On waking, he suffered a heart attack.

Could a dream be powerful enough to kill? Another case history in psychosomatic medicine tells of a middle-aged woman who had worked hard and long to get to the top rungs of the corporate ladder. Even after she got the "perfect" job, she was haunted by fears of failure, and she often awakened in the night, tormented by nightmares of humiliation and professional disgrace. Just a few months after starting in her new job, she became worried about a female co-worker, whom she saw as a threat to all she had gained. She became obsessed with this woman as a threat to her present and future status. One night she sat upright in bed at 3:00 A.M. and cried, "That woman, she finally got me!" Minutes later she was dead. Doctors reported no previous history of heart disease. The circumstances of her death paralleled those of other cases of sudden death triggered by great trauma in waking life.

If a dream can be hazardous to health, not dreaming might actually improve health. This theory has held up when patients with certain physical and mental diseases were deprived of REM sleep, the time of most active dreaming. Among those who improved after REM deprivation were those with depression, schizophrenia, and neurodermatitis, a chronic skin condition. This approach has been tried only on a temporary basis, but physicians are investigating the long-term effects that REM-suppressing drugs may have on the healthy and the ill.

Rewriting dream scripts

If dreams have the power to make us ill, they also have the potential to make us feel better—in mind and in body. Learning to control our dreams may be one way to gain control of our lives, suggests Cartwright. For several years she has been experimenting with ways of rewriting the "scripts" for recurring dreams. "We are convinced that a certain amount of constructive problem-solving goes on in dreams. Whether we can capitalize on this more consistently by 'preprogramming' dreams remains to be seen," she says.

Cartwright's initial studies showed that people handle emotional problems more realistically after dreaming; that is, they become more willing to confront the problem. The research volunteers were presented with a typical problem for young adults: separation (leaving home), sexual guilt (a possible rape scene), or a conflict between work and pleasure (study versus play). Seven hours later the volunteers were asked to resolve the problem. In the interim, some had stayed awake while others slept. Some of the sleepers had not been disturbed; others were awakened during the night to prohibit REM or NREM sleep. The groups that had not slept at all came up with simple Hollywood-style resolutions. Those whose dreams were not interrupted were more likely to acknowledge the realistic dimensions of the problem.

In 1977 Cartwright began studying sixty women who were recently divorced or separated to see how these women might rewrite their dreams to help change their lives. "For the first few months, the dreams were terribly masochistic," she says. "Everything was the woman's fault. She should be punished. She was responsible. The women were depressed when they went to sleep, dreamed depressing dreams and were redepressed when they woke up."

In the second stage, the women denied a loss in their dreams. They dreamed of reconciliation, comforting dreams that made them feel more depressed when they awoke to discover they weren't true. That's when Cartwright and her colleagues intervened to help them "plot" a new dream. "Some wanted to dream about meeting someone new, but the happy endings we hope that they'll concentrate on are things they can do for themselves, like getting a job or starting a new career." One woman kept dreaming of walking along a beach and being swallowed by a giant wave. The dream seemed to indicate that she was being overwhelmed by life and could not cope. The researcher working with her suggested that she try swimming. The next night, she was again swallowed by the wave, but when she popped to the surface, she began swimming. Her nightmare lost its terror and gave her a sense that she could cope with life.

During the experiment, each woman spent several nights at Cartwright's sleep laboratory with a microswitch taped to her palm. When the patient experienced the repetitive dream, she pressed on the switch, which is so sensitive that she did not have to awaken to operate it. The sleep researchers then responded with a tone that acted as a signal for the woman to change the ending of her dream to the happy solution of her choice. "One function of dreams may be to restore our sense of competence," says Cartwright. "The need to restore competence obviously varies: when things are going well, when we have good days, we do not need much restoration; after serious problems or disastrous days, it may take us more than one night to recoup our losses."

As you descend into dream-sleep, you may be preoccupied by a feeling remaining from the previous day, perhaps one of anxiety or depression. This feeling, according to Cartwright, is what motivates the dream and helps select its imagery. Even if you wake up without a succinct solution to your problem, you're better prepared emotionally to cope with the situation. Dreaming seems to modulate the heights of your anxiety or the depths of your depression, so the next day you are not as bogged down with negative feelings.

Dreams also help you recast your self-image. "We often get fragmented during the day about who it is we think we are in the world," says Cartwright. Somebody may say you're not as pretty as you thought you are, or whatever. That night—provided the information wasn't too repetitive during the day—dreaming helps you reconstitute yourself so you can get up intact with your self-picture pretty much restored. Now, if this new information happens to be true—for example, if you're not as pretty as you thought you were, if you've gotten old or fat while you weren't watching—then dreaming tends to incorporate the new information and help you restructure a new self-concept that you can live with."

At the Veterans Administration Hospital in Cincinnati, Milton Kramer's work has provided evidence that dreams can affect mood. Volunteers, awakened at the end of REM sleep on twenty consecutive nights, had their dream reports analyzed and their moods evaluated in the morning. The more people who appeared in the dreams, Kramer found, the more the dreamer's mood improved during the night. Yet dreams themselves are affected by the preceding day's mood. As Kramer explains it, dreams are part of an unbroken chain. Your emotional state influences what you dream—particularly what or whom you dream about—and what you dream influences how you feel the next day. "You don't just have to be the passive observer," says Kramer. "Right before you fall asleep you can focus on the person or persons who make you feel good. That increases the likelihood that they'll turn up in your dreams and make you feel better. We're very social animals. We don't like to be alone in our dreams any more than we like to be alone in the day." Kramer believes that the

The Facts of Sleep

essence of dreams is psychological: "When it comes to dreams, two things are important: meaning and function. Do dreams enlighten us about ourselves? Will they make us smarter, change our personality, change our mood, solve our problems, have any application to our daily lives?" The answer to these questions, according to dream researchers, is an unequivocal yes.

The "stuff" of dreams: mind or matter?

The reports of the dreams that fill our nights are intriguing, but they sidestep a fundamental question: Why are we dreaming at all? Are dreams the arena in which we parade and encounter fears and wishes banished from daytime thoughts? This is what traditional psychologists and psychiatrists might say. But two Harvard psychiatrists—J. Allan Hobson, M.D., and Robert McCarley, M.D.—believe that dreams are caused by stimulation of the brain, and that neurons (nerve cells) and neurotransmitters (messenger chemicals in the brain), not buried memories and pains, are the "stuff" of which dreams are made.

Freud believed that the brain was incapable of producing its own energy and used neurons as reservoirs to store energy from other sources, primarily from sexual and aggressive drives. Arguing that instinctual drives furnish the energy for dreaming, Freud contended that we could understand more about these elemental drives if we understood more about dreams. Psychiatrists created an elaborate system for translating dream symbols: cylindrical objects were phallic symbols, vessels or buildings were female symbols, a feeling of floating reflected the dreamer's view of his or her place in the world.

Could we be interpreting too much from such dream images? According to Hobson and McCarley, dreams may be nothing more than the thinking brain's effort to make sense of confusing signals from the brain regions involved in REM sleep. They view dreams as the psychological accompaniment of biological and chemical changes in the brainstem—as the sideshow rather than the main event.

During twelve years of studying what happens as cats sleep and dream, Hobson and McCarley traced the pathway for dreams, identifying neurons that turn on during REM and others that turn off during dreams. These "giant" nerve cells activated during REM have long "fingers" or tendrils that extend into parts of the brain concerned with eye movement, balance, and repetitive actions such as walking and running. The activated neurons jostle other nerve cells, such as those involved in perception; they, in turn, send messages to the higher regions of the brain. The brain registers the fact that the cells usually involved in walking or watching are turned on, even though the body itself is neither walking nor watching. Struggling to come up with a coherent explanation, the brain flips through various scenes and characters stored in its memory and manufactures a dream.

McCarley compares this process to what goes on in a newsroom during a big story, such as a five-alarm fire. The reporters at the scene call in their reports: one describes the fire; one interviews the fire chief; one does a "human-interest" report on a little boy crying for his lost dog. A "rewrite" editor, sitting miles away in a newsroom desk, puts together the bits and pieces of the story and writes a comprehensive article on the fire. During a dream, the "reporter" cells in the brainstem inform the brain that they are receiving signals to move, but the muscles of movement are inhibited and the body is immobile. The brain has to "rewrite" these reports into a logical story.

Hobson and McCarley have demonstrated that in cats the brain is indeed giving commands during sleep. They destroyed the part of the brain that inhibits muscular activity and then allowed the cats to sleep. During REM, the cats literally acted out their dreams: they leapt into the air, arched their backs, toyed with imaginary mice, and clawed at invisible enemies.

This theory offers a logical explanation for why we so often feel paralyzed in dreams, particularly when endangered. "The brain is being told we are running," says Hobson, "but it is not receiving feedback from the periphery to confirm it. We are unable to move our feet, and that fact is readily communicated." Similarly, we dream of flying because the brain is receiving disparate signals from our ventricular activating, or balance, mechanisms. Eight percent of dream reports describe sensations of floating, flying, or spinning, experiences that do not occur in waking life. The frequency of these sensations in dreams may be due to the fact that the world does seem to move when there are sudden, uncoordinated eye movements, or these images could be influenced by the neurons on those cells that regulate the position and balance of the head and neck.

Why are there so many sudden scene shifts in dreams? Freudians would say the dreamer is trying to avoid unpleasant material. Hobson and McCarley say a shift occurs when different neurons run the course of their activity and another sequence takes over. They also feel that the reason visual sensations are so common in dreams, while almost no one mentions sensations of taste or smell or pain is that fantastic images may be the only way the brain can knit together a vast amount of contradictory information.

This view of dreams has been criticized by followers of more traditional Freudian views, who argue that Hobson and McCarley are trying to reduce dreams to a matter of cellular maneuvers. In their own defense, Hobson and McCarley say that they are not out to undermine conventional psychiatric dream theory and that there is a correlation between their views and those of others. An example of this congruity is a dream report of a man who came upon two people he disliked, who proceeded to spit at him. The dreamer felt a growing desire to spit. Eventually this urge became so overwhelming that he woke up. On waking, he realized that his throat was clogged with mucus and he did indeed have to spit. The urge to spit was real and physical, but it was his dislike for the people in the dream that provided a psychological explanation for his wanting to spit at them. Similarly, men may report more sexual dreams than women because of physical as well as psychological reasons: their brains may be receiving information that the penis is erect and may be drawing on sexual memories or fantasies to explain this phenomenon.

If dreams are as crucial to the brain as they are to the mind, they may be particularly important in maintaining the acuity of that organ. As Hobson explains, "Dreams may be the signals made by the system as it steps through a built-in test pattern—a kind of brain tune-up crucial to prepare the organism for behavioral competence." This new way of thinking about dreams is also important for another reason: it reminds us that mind and body are indeed one and that even in sleep they cannot be separated.

Dreaming your life away

Most people remember only one or two dreams a week, a mere ten percent of their dream-life. Often the reason for forgetting is a matter of bad timing. To remember a dream, you have to wake up within a few minutes of its occurrence. You tend to remember more dreams on weekends because you have the time to try and shift back to sleep to capture a dream fragment. During the week, you may be too busy scurrying into your morning routine to backtrack and recall a memory or a dream image.

It is possible to train yourself to remember your dreams better. At bedtime, tell yourself that you are going to dream and recall your dreams. Keep a pad and pencil by your bed and record your dreams whenever you awaken from them. If you are determined to tune into your dreams, you can set your alarm at two-hour intervals throughout the night so that you are awakened from REM periods, when you are most likely to be dreaming vividly. In the morning, allow yourself time to linger in bed to retain your dream memories. You might want to keep a dream diary to record and find patterns and subtle meanings in your dreams.

You might even try putting your dreams to work on your problems. One psychologist, Gayle Delaney, Ph.D., has developed an approach she calls "dream incubation." Before going to sleep, record the events of the day and a few brief statements about a particular problem you are wrestling with. Next, write in big letters a one-line phrase that asks the question most pertinent to the problem, such as, "What's going on between us?" or "Why do I feel I've come to a dead-end in this relationship?" Repeat the question, over and over like a mantra or lullaby, until sleep comes. Upon awakening, write down whatever comes to your mind, whether it is a dream, a fragment of a dream, an isolated image, or a word from a song. Whatever it is, it is relevant. Then you can try to match up that echo from the night with a person or part of daily life. When it fits together, you will understand how the dream touches your life and your problem.

You can also take a much more casual approach to plugging into your dreams: simply focus on remembering some snatches of your nighttime fantasies. Gradually an understanding of your dreams may lead you to a deeper awareness of your actions and reactions in waking life. Your dreaming mind might be the ideal agent for bringing together the two worlds of night and day. As you see how the two realms merge, you may also discover more about the way in which your fears and fantasies, realities and hopes, memories and expectations come together in your dreams.

CHAPTER 5

The Sleeping Brain

T he sleeping brain is a perceptual paradox. It can "see" without seeing, "hear" without hearing, "feel" without touching. The world your brain conjures up at night is vivid, dynamic, and full, and the links between it and the realities of your daily life are complex.

How are you able to summon up a vast repertoire of stories, complete with lights, action, characters, and plot, as you lie quietly in bed? Is the sleeping brain an internal equivalent of a Hollywood producer, casting dream roles and setting up fantasy scenes? Or is there more serious work going on? Are you assimilating data as you sleep, memorizing what's important and discarding what's not? Does your brain use the hours of the night to work out solutions to the problems and challenges of the day?

These are questions researchers are asking as they explore the complexities of the human brain, the organ that Hippocrates once described as the source of "pleasures, joys, delights, laughter and jests, and sorrows, pains, griefs and tears." But awake or asleep, your brain is the machinery of your mind. The two are intertwined and interdependent. In pioneering studies of the troubled sleep of troubled people, scientists are gaining new insight into underlying mechanisms of mental illness. These investigations of the sleeping brain hold great promise as a means by which we can learn more about ourselves and the machinery of our minds.

Night school

Because it is so difficult to think about the organ of thought, many scientists use analogies to explain the workings of the brain. They particularly like to compare the brain to a computer. All day long data are fed into this highly sophisticated information-processor, and the brain sorts through the new input and determines appropriate responses. What happens at night? Is the plug pulled so that the computer shuts down?

Not at all, say researchers. Sleep—particularly REM sleep—seems to be a critical time for assimilating information. The sleeping brain does more than replay scenes from the day. It integrates what you've learned and helps you to master difficult subjects or tasks. In experiments with laboratory mice, investigators have found that REM or lack of REM makes a difference in the ability of the mice to perform complex tasks. REM did not seem significant in rather straightforward matters, but if the animals did not go into REM sleep *after* learning to differentiate shades of color or to cooperate with each other in a survival test, they forgot their new skills.

Humans may be similar to mice in their need to "sleep on" new material. Some studies have shown that the amount of time in REM sleep is directly correlated with mastery of new and difficult information. For example, University of Ottawa researchers discovered that students who learned quickly in an intensive language course tended to increase their REM time at night, while the slower learners did not. And the students with longer REM periods received better grades. However, sleep researchers have not been able to confirm that this sort of association between learning and sleep is common.

Yet the brain may be involved in more than just "book-learning" at night. People wrestling with complex life issues may need to work out their difficulties by night as well as by day. Could major life changes actually increase the need to sleep and dream? Psychologist Rosalind Cartwright, Ph.D., set out to test this hypothesis by studying thirty women, between the ages of thirty and fifty-five, who were in the midst of separation or divorce proceedings. "We predicted that women with traditional values as well as those with more liberated values, who are emotionally upset during the transition, would have more pressure to dream," she explains. Her early findings supported this premise. The separated and divorced women began REM sleep much earlier in the night than other women, usually in less than an hour. However, many sleep researchers are reluctant to conclude that the earlier onset of REM sleep is only a manifestation of increased REM pressure. The earlier onset may be the result of a phase shift, so that REM occurs earlier in the night but total REM time does not increase.

From infancy to old age, REM seems to be essential for peak performance of our brains and minds. Babies may spend so much time in REM-like active sleep because they have so much to learn about themselves and their world. As adults, we may spend far less time in REM because we have already assimilated the basic data we need to survive. Although we may need less, we definitely need some REM each night. In one study of men and women over the age of sixty-five, those who spent the most time in REM are sharpest in mental responsiveness.

Is there a way to exploit the learning capacity of the sleeping brain? American sleep researchers are skeptical. Since REM is a time of internal processing, the brain is not responsive to new external material. However, certain types of people may be responsive to learning in the "twilight zones" of consciousness, the period of semiwakefulness before sleep. A psychologist at the University of Colorado has suggested that students with mental blocks about certain subjects (like a foreign language) or obese people unable to comply with advice about good eating habits might be more open-minded just before sleep because of a suspension of critical judgment.

The amount of actual learning that is possible seems limited, however. In one experiment, tape-recordings of pairs of English and Russian words were played while the subjects were getting ready for bed. The next morning they were unable to recall any of the pairs unaided and could not correctly respond to Russian words, but they were able to recognize correct word pairings at a rate 15 percent higher than chance. The Russians have reported much greater success in teaching English by night. In one Soviet town, some 1,000 residents allegedly learned English by listening to classes on radio when they went to bed.

All-nighters: sleep and memory

Although sleep may not be a good time for learning new material, it is essential for processing data collected during the day. The beneficial effects of sleep on memory were recognized more than half a century ago when researchers compared the recall of volunteers who slept after memorization with those who stayed awake. Those who slept remembered more. Experiments have since confirmed that sleep aids memory, whether a person sleeps immediately after learning or waits a few hours. In one study, three groups of people learned a word task. One group immediately went to bed for seven hours, another group stayed awake for seven hours and then slept for seven hours, and the third group stayed awake for fourteen hours straight. All three groups were tested fourteen hours after learning the new material. Recall was about the same in the two groups who had slept but was better than for those who stayed awake.

Only sleep that *follows* study helps memory, however. Sleep prior to learning can be worse than no sleep at all, and even a short period of sleep just before learning makes it more difficult to remember the material. In one experiment, subjects slept for a specified period of time and then were given a list of facts to memorize. The researchers made sure the subjects were fully alert before they started, so drowsiness was not a factor. Four hours later the subjects were tested for recall. Prior sleep of half an hour, one hour, two hours, and four hours all impaired memory. But if subjects were awakened two to four hours before learning, their memory was no longer affected by sleep. And if they were allowed to sleep six hours rather than four before learning, they remembered more.

This research may have practical implications for late-night crammers. Sleeping first and waking up early to study before a big test will not help. Even though you may have read the material just hours before the test, you will not be able to recall it well because of the prior sleep effect. Staying up all night is also pointless; you may be too drowsy to perform well.

How does a brief period of sleep erase memory? The hormonal changes associated with different phases of sleep may be responsible. The level of hormone called somatotropin usually rises quickly within thirty minutes of sleep onset and reaches a peak in the first half of the night; the level of somatotropin decreases in the second part of a night's sleep. Laboratory experiments have shown that somatotropin affects memory in mice. The mice were injected with the hormone at various times before and after training and were tested for memory loss four weeks later. When somatotropin was injected five minutes before training, memory was severely disrupted. If it was injected ninety minutes before training, there was no significant difference in recall from those mice who had not been injected with the hormone. If somatotropin works the same way in humans, people awakened early in sleep may experience poor recall because of the hormone's high level of activity. Somatotropin levels gradually return to normal after awakening, which may account for the disappearance of the prior-sleep effect after a subject has been awake for a while after brief sleep.

The round-the-clock surges of hormones may indicate that there is a circadian or daily rhythm in our memories as well as our glands. In one experiment, researchers tried to distinguish the effects of sleep and the timing of sleep on recall. Those who slept at night remembered more than those who slept during the day. The daytime sleepers forgot just as much as those who did not sleep at all. The biochemical and hormonal changes that usually occur during sleep at night may preclude assimilation of new material. This may be why you do not remember phone calls in the night or why you forget your dreams. The brain may not be capable of receiving and processing this information during sleep.

Night vision

While the body rests at night, the sensory apparatus of the brain does not rest. You continue to see and to hear in your dreams as you sleep. Does the way you see and hear things by day affect these nighttime perceptions? To answer this question, researchers decided to change the way a group of volunteers looked at the world around them. All day during the course of the experiment they viewed their environment through red-colored goggles. When awakened while dreaming at night, they reported the reddish hue in their dreams. Regardless of whether the dreams included daytime images or childhood memories, they appeared in shades of red. Trees and other green objects appeared black, as they did when viewed through the red goggles during the day. Even the most fantastic visions were shaded in red.

In further experiments on the links between waking perception and sleep images, researchers at the University of Texas designed elaborate "mini-faction" goggles. Looking through these multiple-gadgeted glasses is similar to looking through binoculars the wrong way. When volunteers wear the computer-monitored lenses, the researchers can determine whether restrictions on eye movements in the awake state affect eye movements in REM sleep.

Initial findings have not shown a strong correlation between the actual movements of the eyes during the awake state and during sleep, but the dream images of the volunteers did become distorted. Additional evidence has indicated an association between what we see by day and what we dream by night. For example, several studies have shown that people who were born blind have dreams filled with sounds rather than sights; only those who once were sighted have visual dreams.

Sound is usually secondary in dreams, but our ears are active in the night. The muscles of the middle ear, which respond to loud sound during waking, vibrate before and during REM periods. Approximately 80 percent of nightly ear activity occurs during REM and the rest occurs immediately before or after it. Middle ear muscular activity (MEMA), like rapid eye movement, is not continuous or synchronized. A loud noise will trigger greater activity. A dreamer awakened by a sudden sound during REM sleep may incorporate it into the dream story and report an explosion or crash in the dream.

The eyes and ears are so involved in dreaming that researchers question what would happen to our daytime perception of sights or sounds if we could not dream. In the longest marathons of wakefulness, frightening hallucinations and perceptional distortions have been reported. When radio disc jockey Peter Tripp stayed awake for almost ten days, he saw flames blazing in a desk drawer, clocks with human faces, and specks that turned into bugs.

As demonstrated in sleep laboratory experiments, REM deprivation definitely increases the pressure to enter REM sleep. The sleepers become more difficult to awaken from REM and the intervals between nighttime REM periods grow shorter, as does the time from sleep onset to the first signs of REM. When awake, some REM-deprived people have shown anxiety, irritability, and problems in concentrating. However, there is no evidence that prolonged REM deprivation will cause dreams to erupt into the waking state either in sleep attacks (similar to those of a narcoleptic) or in hallucinations. There seems to be a powerful barrier that prevents REM from spilling into our waking consciousness.

But once REM-deprived people are allowed to sleep through the night, there are dramatic differences in their sleep patterns, and they spend much more time than usual in REM. This sort of REM rebound also occurs after REM has been suppressed by alcohol or drugs. The dreams of a drinker or drug user in withdrawal are often bizarre and frightening, while the volunteers in REM-deprivation experiments rarely report such dreams.

In cats, REM deprivation has more dramatic effects: the animals seem to lose control of their various appetites. They act uncontrollably hungry. They become hypersexual, and some male cats even mount anesthetized or dead animals. A person showing such loss of control might well be considered mentally deranged, perhaps dangerously so. The lack of REM, not just the lack of sleep, may explain the bizarre perceptual and behavioral changes that Peter Tripp experienced when he tried to live without sleep.

Troubled minds, troubled nights

Some people have long suggested that in the dreams of night we flirt with madness. The daytime world of a psychotic is often described as being as bizarre as a dream, and one theory about the purpose of dreams is that they are the outlet for impulses that might otherwise drive us mad. The relationship of sleep, dreams, and mental illness is much more complex, however, and psychiatrists and psychologists are finding clues to the problems of the mind by studying changes in the processes of the sleeping brain.

Sleep problems and mental disturbances are considered clinical bedfellows. Difficulty in sleeping is often the first complaint of those troubled by emotional or mental problems. Sleep disorders may be universal in those who suffer from depression, a complaint so common in our society that it is considered to be the mental equivalent of the common cold.

Everyone experiences times of sadness or discouragement; these may be the appropriate responses to particular life events. Psychiatrists refer to feelings triggered by external events, such as the loss of a loved one, personal failure, or physical illness, as "reactive" depression. "Endogenous" depression rises from within and is much more complex. While sadness may be a symptom, it is far from the only one. Such depression affects a person in many subtle ways and may lead to a loss of appetite and weight, loss of sexual drive, neglect of appearance and hygiene, "palpitations" or flutters of the heart, shortness of breath, poor memory, an inability to concentrate, indecisiveness, feelings of guilt, illogical thought processes, and withdrawal from others. In its severe and chronic forms, depression can be a life-threatening illness.

In order to learn more about this complex disorder, scientists are studying the way people with certain types of depression spend the night. They have found that depressed people enter REM sleep much earlier in the night than normal, their sleep is not continuous, their NREM sleep is less deep, and the number of eye movements per minute of REM sleep is increased. The most significant of these characteristics seems to be the shortened time between sleep onset and REM, a period called REM latency. While a normal person spends 80 to 110 minutes asleep before dreaming, a depressed person enters REM within five to forty minutes. It may be that the more severe the depression, the shorter REM latency becomes. In studies at the University of Pittsburgh, psychiatrist David Kupfer, M.D., and his colleagues have been studying REM latency in the depressed as a possible biological marker of this mental illness and a means of diagnosing it more accurately. This could lead to a major advance in determining appropriate and effective treatment plans.

Since REM latency varies with age, researchers have studied the normal sleep patterns of the very young and the elderly and have compared them to the disordered sleep patterns of the depressed. They've found that while sixty-five-year-olds normally enter REM sleep earlier than twenty-five-year-olds, depressed sixty-five-year-olds have an even shorter REM latency. Depressed children or teenagers have a longer REM latency than that of adults but one that is considerably shorter when compared to the sleep patterns of their peers.

Several groups of scientists have wondered whether the disrupted sleep patterns of the depressed may be signs of a disturbance in the brain's circadian rhythms. A short REM latency and a concentration of REM sleep in the early part of the night, rather than in the second half, may be a symptom of such disharmony. According to one theory, an underlying cause of depression may be a damaged or weakened sleep-cycle "oscillator" or pace-setter. If so, resetting this internal clock might help the problems of the brain's cycling and the mind's depression.

Various experiments have tested this theory. REM deprivation, for example, seemed to stimulate the REM sleep control system and lift depression—but only temporarily. After REM deprivation, the depressed volunteers slept more normally; that is, they dreamed later in the night. At the National Institute of Mental Health, scientists tried another approach: "phase-advancing" depressed patients. They moved their bedtimes from the usual 11:00 P.M. to 5:00 P.M., and they woke them up at 1:00 A.M. rather than 7:00 A.M. The patients who slept on this schedule still dreamed at approximately the same time (midnight), but REM occurred in the second half of their "night." The treatment worked in that the depressed patients felt better—but again only for a little while. Their REM rhythm eventually shifted so that they were again dreaming soon after they fell asleep. A second phase-advance was effective, but a third was not. "We changed the world's schedule around the patients to fix their rhythms," explains researcher Thomas Wehr, M.D. "The next step is finding a way to fix the rhythms to suit the world, either by speeding them up or slowing them down." He believes that manipulating external time cues could influence the circadian timing of REM sleep.

The questions these scientists are asking are fundamental. They want to understand why some people fail to respond to the stimuli that keep us in touch with night and day. Interestingly, volunteers who have been removed from all time cues and placed in isolation for extended periods seem to develop the same sleep-wake rhythms as depressed patients. They had longer day-night cycles, short REM latencies, and more intense eye movements during the first REM period. If investigators can figure out why the same changes occur in people isolated from time cues and in those who fail to respond to time cues, they might be closer to understanding the biological nature of depression.

Such research also may lead to a better understanding of treatments for depression. The drugs most commonly used in this disorder—the tricyclics—usually do not produce any benefits for several weeks. The first sign that a drug will be helpful is a lengthening of REM latency; the medication may reset the REM cycle to normal, and other functions may gradually become synchronized with it.

Eventually scientists may be able to use studies of REM latency to determine not only which drugs may help a patient but which persons may be most susceptible to developing certain types of depression. National Institute of Mental Health researchers have used drugs that mimic brain chemicals to produce earlier REM periods in volunteers. Awakened from this chemically triggered sleep, they reported dreams indistinguishable from normal ones. But certain people responded more dramatically than others and had extremely short REM latencies. This supersensitivity seemed to characterize those people who were depressed, had been depressed, or had a family history of depression.

Investigators are looking for similar sleep signs that may lead to better diagnosis and treatment of a less common, severe mental illness, schizophrenia. Soon after REM sleep was identified in the 1950s, sleep researcher William Dement began studying sleep in schizophrenics and found no remarkable differences in their eye movements, although they were less likely than normal patients to remember their dreams. When they did remember them, they described stark scenes with strangers and isolated objects apparently hanging motionless in space. However gripping their daytime hallucinations were, their nightly dreams were bland.

Experiments with REM deprivation in schizophrenics have led to some intriguing findings. Unlike normal subjects, the schizophrenics with acute symptoms had no REM rebound during their first night of uninterrupted sleep, while those in remission did. Yet, acute schizophrenics deprived of REM have shown improvement. In one experiment at the Georgia Mental Institute, five chronic schizophrenics were deprived of REM for seven nights. Before the experiment, all had acute symptoms, including hallucinations, delusions, and assaultive behavior. During the REM-less period, none had any such episodes.

Continuing research may lead to more accurate ways of diagnosing schizophrenia. At Stanford University, psychiatrist Vincent Zarcone, M.D., has documented differences in the activity of the middle ear muscles (MEMs) in schizophrenics and normal people. "The diagnosis of schizophrenia may be made too often for too many problems in too many people," he says. "Because the implications of having schizophrenia are so serious, an objective means of evaluation would be very significant." The use of sleep science to supply such tools for understanding brains and minds is relatively recent. However, the study of the sleeping brain may provide many more clues for those trying to figure out the intricate puzzles—and problems—of the human mind.

The secret life of neurons

Even the brains of the most brilliant people have a frustrating limitation: they cannot explain themselves. This is why the brain is the least understood organ, why it is so difficult to use the brain to comprehend the brain. Only recently have neuroscientists developed methods for unlocking the mysteries of the mind, for discovering the complexities of the millions of neurons within the 3½-pound lump of grayish tissue that is the human brain. Sleep research is one of the means that scientists are using to peer within this fascinating organ.

The intensity of activity within the sleeping brain has yielded clues as to its nature and needs. The discharge of electrical impulses from neurons during REM may be a built-in source of stimulation for the brain, reflecting its relentless and basic need to fill itself with thought. "A stimulated nerve cell, especially in a developing human or animal, is a happy nerve cell," says Howard Roffwarg, M.D., of the University of Texas. "When there's no stimulation, the cells shrivel up and stop working normally." The orderly progression of REM and NREM periods during the night may force the brain to use the faculties essential for waking life. REM may serve its most vital function early in life, when the fetus and newborn spend much of their time in a state of active sleep. During this REM-like period, the internal activity of the brain may aid in the process by which the nervous system matures. Child development specialists have offered evidence to support this theory: babies with genetic mental abnormalities spend less time in active sleep than normal, healthy infants.

By studying the chemical properties of sleep, scientists may be able to trace the pathways by which the brain's cells communicate with each other and with other parts of the body. Eventually such research might yield better under-standing of the diseases that can occur when even a few of our billions of neurons stop working as they should. But before scientists can hope to find cures for such problems, they will need to learn much more about the world within the skull. For years to come, the exploration of the brain, while we are asleep as well as awake, will remain one of the most exciting and important frontiers of science.

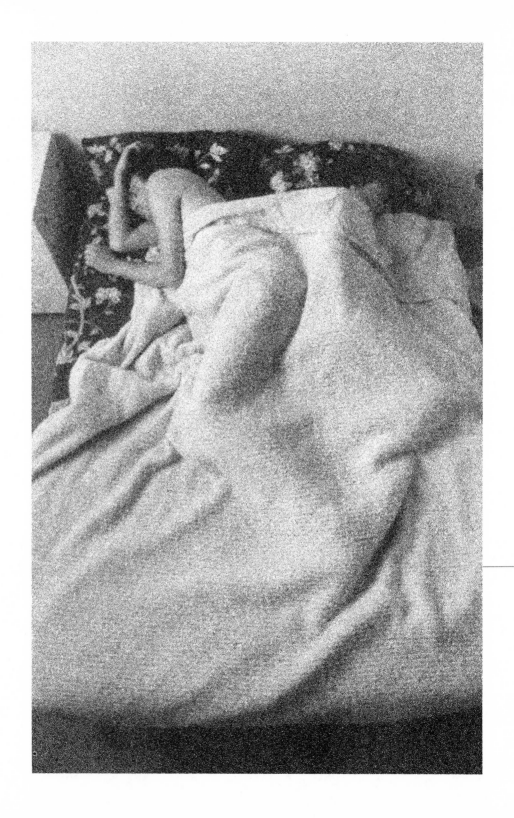

Sleep Sense

CHAPTER 6

Sleep Settings: Rocking Your Cradle

Y our bedroom is your fortress against an intrusive world, your last bastion of privacy. Alone in bed, you can cry into your pillow, pound the mattress, sing, reflect, remember. The rest of your house is for the many strangers who trek through your life and rooms; your bedroom is for a select few. Going to bed with a person has become synonymous with sexual intimacy. Sharing a bed and a bedroom requires mutual trust and consideration. No other place, no other room, reveals more about who you are—or has a greater impact on how you sleep.

If you needed to, you probably could sleep anywhere. Soldiers have slept upright in trenches; travelers on early sailing ships slept on hard, narrow berths; mountain climbers have slept when secured by ropes on rocky ledges. But under less-than-dire circumstances, you need comfort and security. Sleep is a time of vulnerability, and you sleep better when you feel safe and sheltered. Your bedroom is the cradle for your nights, and everything in it—from the bed to curtains to decorations—should soothe you when you lie down to rest. You spend more time in your bedroom than any other room in your house. It is well worth your time to design a place of peace, privacy, and comfort.

The way they slept: the evolution of the bedroom

Other primates, such as the monkeys and apes, rely on the comfort and protection of each other through the night. The first bed invented by man was probably no more than a pile of leaves, covered by an animal hide. Caves were the first "bedrooms," where families snuggled together in the dark. In many developing countries and in the poor communities of industrialized nations, families still sleep together at night. Anthropologists have argued that middle-class American parents, who exile their children to separate beds at birth, are the exception to generations of communual sleeping.

Beds as we know them did not exist in ancient times. Queen Esther's bed was described in the Bible as luxurious, but it was no more than a pile of cushions on the floor. More conventional beds consisted of low tables with wooden headrests. The noble and wealthy eventually devised more ornate places to lay their heads. Egypt's young King Tutankhamen had an exquisite bed of ebony and gold. Babylonian and Assyrian lords slept on bronze beds encrusted with jewels. Nero, emperor of Rome, used precious stones with beneficial powers to adorn his bed. Other Romans preferred cradle-shaped beds with two chambers, one filled with water and the other covered by a mattress. First, they would lie in warm water, rocked by a servant, until they became drowsy; then they'd move onto the mattress and be rocked to sleep.

While peasants of the Middle Ages slept on pallets of straw, their rulers spent more money on building and decorating their beds than on any other piece of furniture. Most popular were canopied beds with rich, thick hangings (which kept the sleeper warm in a drafty castle). Some of these beds were gigantic, and special staircases had to be built for the sleeper to climb into them. The famous Great Bed of Ware in England was 12 feet square and stood 7½ feet off the ground. The household bed was often the most prized legacy passed down through the generations.

During the seventeenth-century reign of Louis XIV, the "Sun King" of France, bedrooms became public places. Louis reportedly owned more than 400 ornate beds and held audiences and supervised state proceedings from them. As French aristocrats imitated him, entertaining from bed became commonplace. Beds grew more and more elaborate, often being equipped with built-in heaters and other luxuries.

Throughout history, bedrooms have been the scene for every human drama, not simply births and deaths. More murders have been committed in bedrooms than in all other rooms combined. Some of the greatest works of music, art, and literature were created in bed, including John Milton's *Paradise Lost*, Charles Darwin's *Origin of the Species*, and many of the writings of Elizabeth Barrett Browning, Edith Wharton, and Colette.

Some famous people have developed fetishes about beds. Vincent van Gogh would sleep only on a pillow made of hops. Benjamin Franklin insisted on having four beds in his room so he could switch to a fresh one whenever a bed became too warm. Charles Dickens rearranged every bedroom he stayed in so that the top of the bed was pointing north. Lawrence of Arabia gave up beds at an early age and slept only in a sleeping bag. Some of the wealthiest and most well-known people in our own society have directed their empires from their bedrooms, including the Baron de Rothschild and Hugh Hefner.

The way we sleep: bedrooms for all reasons

People used to retreat to their bedrooms to get away from it all. Now they may take it all with them. The contemporary bedroom has become more than a place to sleep: it's the hub of a new lifestyle.

Interior decorators talk about the "liberation" of the contemporary bedroom, as if its emergence into the light of day were an occasion of triumph. It is true that many bedrooms are being used around the clock. Today's bedroom may contain not only a bed and bureau but also a desk, files, exercise equipment, a television, a library, a refrigerator (conveniently tucked into a nightstand), stereo system, and most recently, a home computer. The *New York Times* notes that most major cities are filled "with hard-working fast-rising professional couples whose private lives revolve around the bedroom. At the end of the daily rat race, these couples want nothing so much as to collapse in their bedrooms, gathering strength for tomorrow's race."

Childless couples—and there are more than ever before—may prefer the intimacy of the bedroom to the family-sized dimensions of other rooms. If both partners work, they don't have time to whip up elaborate meals in the kitchen, host elegant dinner parties in the dining room, or invite neighbors for cocktails in the living room. These family and public rooms have become, as one social scientist puts it, "places of passage." In the most private and personal of places—the bedroom—each partner talks, reads, eats, listens to music, watches television, balances the checkbook, exercises, makes phone calls, and attends to miscellaneous chores. Sometimes there is literally no other space available. With apartment rents and housing costs skyrocketing, couples and families may need to use every room in the house for dual purposes: bed and desk may end up side by side.

Sociologists worry about such invasions of the bedroom—and so do sleep therapists. When you bring business into the bedroom, the behaviors, attitudes, and burdens of the workaday world usually tag along. The bedroom begins to sound and feel, if not look, like a boardroom. "Instead of a place to retire and enjoy one another intimately," notes sociologist Jeffrey Goldfarb of the New School for Social Research in New York City, "the bedroom is becoming a place where people ignore one another. . . . Already the bedroom is a place to turn off; that's what turning on the television is all about. When it becomes a place to transact business, it will be less likely a place to make love."

It may also be a less likely place for good sleep. All the pressures of the day, including files, reports, and memos, may be neither out of sight nor out of mind. Like crumbs from a chocolate cake nibbled in the night, reminders of daytime responsibilities may creep between the sheets.

When a multi-purpose bedroom is a necessity, some people try to subdivide it for various functions. Some decorators have designed activity modules for the bedroom: one unit includes a desk, shelves, and files; another houses the entertainment systems, including stereo and video; the bed and its accessories are tucked into another place. Such lines of demarcation are critical. Even a simpler barrier, like a divider-bookshelf, may help maintain a clear distinction between the places of work and sleep. Some sleepers are even choosing beds with curtains and canopies, reminiscent of the Middle Ages, to create an aura of seclusion.

If you do use your bedroom for work or exercise or other projects, try to maintain some psychological as well as physical distance. Tell yourself that after you finish, you are going to relax and then go to bed. Use this thought to condition yourself to think of your evening activity as a prelude to sleep. Whenever you must bring work into the bedroom, keep it out of bed. Stake out a part of the room that will remain an exclusively nocturnal preserve. And develop a ritual that will make the transition from daytime preoccupations to bed and sleep more than a journey of several yards.

Finding the bed that's best for you

Even when reminders of daily life pile up around you, your bed should remain a sanctuary. Since you'll spend more time on your bed than on any other piece of furniture, you should choose it carefully. Today there are more varieties of beds available than ever before. But as Goldilocks discovered in the fairytale, some beds can be too big or too hard, some too small or too soft. Shop around to make sure you get a bed that's just right for you.

Size

Size is the first consideration. Will a single bed suffice? Is a double bed big enough for two? If you get a king-size bed, will you feel stranded during the night?

Pop psychologists theorize that any adult who buys a single bed is sending a message: "Leave me alone." The buyer of a three-quarters bed may be hedging; the double-bed owner wants an intimate relationship; the king-size-bed purchaser needs a lot of space. However, you don't buy a bed to make a statement, so concentrate on getting the one that best suits your needs.

In general, your bed should be at least six inches longer than you are and should be large enough for you to move comfortably from side to side. If you are going to share a bed, you should shop for it with your bed partner. Lie down side by side; roll over; extend your arms. The longer or larger you are, the more bed space you need. Remember that each person on a double bed has only as much space as in a crib. If you want something larger, even king-size beds come in alternate sizes: the standard king-size bed is eighty inches long and seventy-six inches wide; a California king-size bed is eighty-four inches long and seventy-two inches wide.

Should you get a bed big enough for two or sleep your separate ways at night? That depends on how you sleep. If one person snores heavily or moves often in the night, the other may want to get out of striking or hearing range. You are not likely to be very tolerant when awakened by a sharp kick or a serenade of snores. It's better to separate the mattresses than end the relationship.

Mattress matters

The ideal mattress cradles the spine so that it maintains the same shape as a person with good upright posture, with the chin, stomach, and pelvis tucked in. If you sleep on a mattress that is too hard or too soft, your muscles must work constantly to straighten your spine. The tug-of-war between mattress and muscle can interfere with your sleep and leave you with a morning backache. According to the American Academy of Orthopedic Surgeons, inadequate support through the night, coupled with poor posture, lack of exercise, and sudden stress, accounts for the periodic backaches suffered by half the population over age twenty-five and virtually everyone over forty-five. An estimated nine million Americans have chronic back problems; the wrong mattress can add considerably to their woes.

A good mattress and box spring will last ten to fifteen years; cheaper ones may wear out in just a few years. Your body will give you the first clue that you need a new mattress. If you wake up wincing, look at the mattress. Are there obvious troughs and ridges? Are there lumps? Has a spring broken through? Do you set off a small dust storm if you hit it? Is the stitching loose or the ticking ripped? When you lie down, does the mattress swallow your body? Sit on the edge and stand up quickly. Does the mattress bounce back into shape? If your mattress is starting to sag, a bed board (usually three-quarter-inch plywood) may work temporarily. However, if the mattress is thick and soft, a bed board will limit but will not eliminate the sag. And a droop of only two inches can cause back problems.

The major alternatives to consider in choosing a new mattress are as follows:

INNERSPRING MATTRESSES: These are the conventional mattresses available in any department or bedding store. They range in price from $150 for a twin mattress and foundation to more than $600 for a king-size set. Ask to see sample construction charts for several different mattresses. A tufted mattress will retain its shape and sag less quickly than one with a smooth surface. Quilting is recommended, but design is irrelevant. Look for an innerspring mattress with a coil count of at least 300 for every fifty-four inches of mattress. Check for squeaks and buoyancy by lying on it; check for support in the areas where body weight is concentrated. The edges may be the best clue as to how well the mattress is made; they should be sturdy and firm. Also check for ventilation holes, and handles for easy moving.

FOAM MATTRESSES: Generally, the thicker a foam mattress, the firmer it is. And the heavier the foam the better, because the denser mattress will have fewer air bubbles and will be less likely to disintegrate. The most common ingredient in foam mattresses is urethane, an oil-based product that can cause intense allergic reactions in some people. The best and most expensive type of foam is latex. Foam prices range from $50 for one that will wear out quickly to $300 for a more durable mattress. Some people stack six-inch or eight-inch pads on each other for more support.

WATERBEDS: Three thousand years ago Persians slept on goatskins filled with water, but it wasn't until 1967 that a California student designed the modern waterbed. At first, sleeping on a water bed was seen as a fad for the young, eccentric, or sexually experimental; now waterbeds have become popular with all types of sleepers.

There is much more to a waterbed than a bag of water. The standard package includes a safety liner (to catch any leaks), frame, heater, and platform or pedestal. Nearly all waterbeds are seven feet long and five or six feet wide. The cost of a waterbed begins at $300 and rises according to the thickness of the vinyl (twenty to twenty-four millimeters), the type of seam construction, and the frame. The most expensive waterbeds have "waveless" lap-seamed construction with interior baffles (barriers) that impede the motion of the water.

Many waterbed owners say that they wouldn't sleep on anything else. Because of the heater beneath the water, this type of mattress can help keep you warm in winter and, without the heater, cool in summer. Leaks have become less of a problem because of recent improvements in the vinyl construction. And although waterbeds are heavy (the king-size bed contains 235 gallons; the queen-size, 196), they're easily emptied and moved. Doctors are divided about the health benefits of these beds, which are used routinely for patients with burns or bedsores. A California orthopedic surgeon who tested four types of mattresses found that a standard waterbed provides the most even distribution of support for the entire body. However, others claim that waterbeds form contours according to body weight rather than structure and are bad for the back because the buttocks sink into the bed and cause the lower back to arch.

How to buy a bed

Once you decide on the size and type of mattress you want, plan to do some serious shopping—on your back as well as your feet:

1 ♦ Dress in comfortable, loose clothing. The only way to try out a bed is to lie

on it. If two people are going to share a bed, they both should shop for it and lie down on it, side by side.

2 ◆ Don't believe that a mattress is "ultra-firm" because a tag says so. Such terms are advertising adjectives, not scientific assessments. Only your body can tell you whether one mattress feels firmer than another.

3 ◆ Don't buy a mattress on the basis of an endorsement by a medical group. These endorsements occasionally are based on testing, but sometimes they are based on more superficial agreements. And whatever the seal of approval, there's no one mattress that is right for everyone.

4 ◆ Don't just lie down on a bed and hop off. If you've been on your feet shopping, any mattress will feel good initially. Stay on the bed for five or ten minutes to see if it continues to be comfortable. Roll over on your side. Stretch. Make sure that you will have enough room to move.

5 ◆ If you and your bed partner cannot agree on the right firmness or size, consider separate beds or twin beds that share one box spring or platform.

6 ◆ Roll to the edge of the bed. It should support you and should not sag. Droopy edges are a sure giveaway of a poorly constructed mattress.

7 ◆ To check on how well the mattress will support you, push down with your hips and shoulders. The mattress should push back firmly but with some resilience.

8 ◆ It is always best to buy a new mattress and box springs as a set. A "sleep set" of mattress and foundation designed to be used together should offer maximum support and wear.

9 ◆ You get what you pay for in mattresses. Consider the fact that your bed will get more use than any other piece of furniture in your house, and spend what you can afford for a quality mattress.

10 ◆ Just in case your new bed doesn't feel as comfortable when you take it home, ask about a "comfort guarantee" that will allow you to exchange beds within four weeks of purchase. Make sure such offers are made in writing and find out if there will be charges for the extra pickup and delivery.

Once you get your mattress home, be sure to slip it from side to side and end to end once a month for the first three months and twice a year thereafter. Less expensive mattresses should be turned more often to let air out and prevent lumps.

Tucking yourself in: feather pillows and rainbow sheets

Just as a mattress should support your body in the same posture as if you were standing upright, a pillow should support your head so that it is in the same relation to your shoulders and spine as if you were standing. If the pillow is too thick, your neck muscles will be strained; it it's too soft, your head will sink, and you will feel overheated and uncomfortable. Although most pillows are rectangular, more sleepers are choosing other shapes, including circles, cylinders, and triangles. A popular model is crescent-shaped and does not bunch up when you turn.

The best—and most costly—pillows are made of goose down. Most feather pillows include feathers from ducks, chickens, and turkeys. The costs of feather pillows range from $50 to $100; they should last twenty-five years. Less expensive pillows are made of synthetic materials; people allergic to feathers and animal dander can sleep on none other than these. The best synthetic pillows are made of "continuous multifilament fiber," which is spun into the casing and is available in various degrees of firmness. The prices start at $15; synthetic pillows should last five to seven years.

Once upon a time all pillowcases and sheets were white. Modern designers have splashed a rainbow of colors over contemporary bedclothes. You can sleep on purple, pink, plaid, paisley, or print sheets made of linen, cotton, silk, satin, or synthetics. The total effect can be more colorful than Jackson Pollack's palette.

Some people have worried that all this visual variety may be too stimulating for the sleeper. However, it is unlikely that the colors of sheets affect what goes on behind closed eyelids during sleep. But colors do have an undeniable impact on mood—before and after sleep as well as during the day. Many troubled sleepers prefer the soothing colors of blue and green; some find it easier to wake up in bright, sunshine-colored sheets. Choose whatever colors and patterns make you feel relaxed and comfortable. While silk or satin sheets may seem like the ultimate in sensuality, you may find them distracting if you are not accustomed to them; they also need special care and laundering. Whatever fabric you choose for your sheets, make sure they are clean and smooth. Don't tuck the top sheet in so tightly that you cannot move freely, and don't clutter up the bed with more pillows than you actually use.

You'll probably change the number of blankets and quilts you use with the seasons. Many people, preferring warmth without heaviness, choose electric blankets or down-filled comforters. Others prefer to snuggle beneath a pile of blankets or an old-fashioned quilt. Again, choose whatever suits you best.

With so many available fashions for the bedroom, you may be tempted to turn your bedroom into a scene for a magazine spread. But remember that your bedroom is for you, not for public display. When you decorate, choose items that evoke positive, pleasurable feelings. Photographs of friends that bring back happy memories are fine; pictures of ex-spouses or deceased parents may trigger sudden sadness at bedtime. Pastel watercolors or prints make eye-pleasing wall decorations for a bedroom; surrealist scenes or circus posters should be placed in another room. If you like a sense of order and control, keep your bedroom uncluttered and austere. If you want to indulge in your softer side, fill it with frilly, ruffled curtains and accessories. Don't worry about what your bedroom says about you; let it *be* you.

◆　◆　◆

"Reading" Your Bedroom to Find Out What It Says About You

A bedroom is a reflection of your personality, fantasies, and needs. No matter how it is decorated, it holds clues to the owner's personality. Like a dream, nothing in it is without meaning. Reading a bedroom—your own or someone else's—doesn't require any special skill, just observation and a little common sense. Start with a tour of your own bedroom and see what it says about you:

* *The room is obviously used for: (a) sleeping, (b) retreat, (c) day-to-day living.*
* *The color on the walls inspires one to: (a) lie down and relax, (b) leap up immediately and get something done, (c) shield one's eyes.*
* *The light in the room most closely resembles: (a) early morning in a garden, (b) high noon in the Mojave Desert, (c) soft twilight, (d) midnight in a cave.*
* *On the walls there are: (a) photographs of you and company, (b) framed geometric shapes in primary colors, (c) rhetoric under glass, (d) Nada.*
* *The bed is obviously designed for: (a) sleeping, (b) fun and frolic, (c) day-to-day activities.*

- *It is big enough to hold: (a) just you, thanks, (b) you and a friend, (c) you, a friend, and the rest of the gang.*
- *On it is: (a) a soft, comfortable bedspread, (b) something starched, slick, or bumpy, (c) fur.*
- *On top of that are: (a) three pillows always arranged at right angles to each other, (b) nice, fluffy pillows to lean against, (c) your stuffed animal.*
- *This is obviously the province of: (a) One Hell of a Women, (b) The Sheik of Araby, (c) an innocent bystander.*
- *Your own personality: (a) pervades the room, (b) is expressed in a controlled sort of way, (c) Who?*
- *Someone coming to visit might think: (a) When did the earthquake hit?, (b) Oh God, I invaded your privacy, sorry, excuse me, I'll get out right away!, (c) Whose room did you say this was?, (d) Oh, what a pleasant place. Think I'll stay for a while.*

Courtesy **MADEMOISELLE**. Copyright 1980 by The Condé Nast Publications Inc. Reprinted with permission.

◆   ◆   ◆

Setting the temperature for sleep

The bed that seemed so cozy at bedtime may feel like an oven hours later. You fling off the covers—only to awaken a little later shivering and reaching for the extra blanket.

This is a common scene, the result of normal changes in your body temperature during sleep and of setting the thermostat either too high or low. Most people sleep best in a room that is somewhat cool: 64° to 66°F. The temperature of the air—not whether it is fresh, outdoor air—affects both how long and how well you sleep. If the temperature is much cooler, you will stay in bed longer. If it is much warmer, you will sleep less and toss more.

You can, however, adjust to almost any sleep temperature. Studies at Kansas State University showed that people sleep just as well at 90° as at 50°F—once they adjust to one temperature. This adjustment usually takes a few nights. The simplest solution to staying warm at night is to wear something warm and pile on another blanket. In very cold weather, an electric blanket *under* the sheet can keep you particularly cozy. Because indoor air tends to become very dry in the winter, you might want to buy a humidifier to make breathing more comfortable.

In hot weather, air-conditioning can keep you cool. However, many people dislike the sound of the machine or the quality of the air and prefer a fan. Even on the warmest night, a top sheet will make you feel more comfortable than no covers at all. A cool compress over your forehead and eyes at bedtime may be soothing; a cold shower may be counterproductive because it will signal your body to produce more heat. A tepid bath will feel cool and will help you relax.

Night noise

Quiet is essential to deep, restful sleep. The noise of a jet overhead or a motorcycle backfiring beneath your window may not actually awaken you, but it will disturb your sleep by forcing you to shift from deep sleep into a lighter sleep stage. Sensitivity to noise varies in different individuals, and women are more likely than men to awaken because of noise. Older people, who spend less time in deep sleep, will awaken because of a noise that a child or younger adult will sleep through.

Our ears seem to be sensitive to specific sounds in sleep. A sleeper is more likely to react to a "relevant" sound than to a vague noise. For example, a doctor and his wife, parents of a new baby, reported that they woke up for different sounds in the night: the doctor awakened to the sound of his beeper, but his wife did not; the wife awakened when the baby cried, but the doctor did not.

Contrary to popular belief, people do not adjust to continuous sounds in the night. Studies of residents near Los Angeles airport, for example, showed that they consistently woke up more frequently, spent more time in lighter sleep stages, and had less deep NREM and less REM sleep.

In another study at North Carolina State University, volunteers exposed to thirty-two different sounds in the night generally remembered only two or three. However, sleep recordings revealed that they did shift to lighter sleep. Volunteers who were exposed to twenty-second periods of overhead jet sounds nine times a night experienced significant changes in sleep patterns. The next morning the volunteers couldn't perform a simple task as well as they did after an uninterrupted night. A total of three minutes of aircraft noise disturbed sleep patterns for as long as forty-five minutes. The effect of the noise was far longer than the duration of the sound.

Traffic sounds have a similar effect. A Canadian study showed that passing trucks caused sleepers either to awaken or shift into lighter sleep. Even after two weeks of exposure to traffic noise, sleepers still shifted into lighter sleep, although they were less likely to awaken.

Any sound over seventy decibels begins to stimulate signals from the nervous system to the rest of the body. If the sound is sudden, uninterrupted, and meaningless, the blood pressure increases and the supply of blood to the heart is lowered. As the intensity increases, the pupils dilate, the muscles of the abdomen and chest contract, and the heart rate quickens. (The chart on page 80 shows the decibel levels for some sounds that may arouse you from sleep.)

For the sake of your ears and your sleep, you may want to take defensive measures. Ear plugs can block out noise, but be sure they fit properly so that they don't damage your ears. They may feel uncomfortable at first, but you will adapt. There also are a number of devices that provide unusual sorts of lullabies to help you sleep. "White noise" generators are widely sold. White noise is a sound involving all frequencies audible to the human ear. It lulls the mind because there's no message in this medium; it sounds like your car does when you travel down the freeway at fifty-five miles per hour. The frequency of the sound is less important than its repetition. An air-conditioner set at "fan" also makes a "white noise" sound. Doctors have reported that such devices seem particularly effective in helping babies sleep—especially when the sound is moderately loud.

Some people prefer records or tapes of natural sounds: waterfalls, birds, waves crashing on the shore. If you start listening to one of these tapes every night as you relax or exercise, it could be an effective "cue" for making you sleepy. One record consists of nothing more than the steady thump-thump-thump of a human heart. For an even more womblike experience, there's a shell made of plastic and wood that stretches over the bed and turns it into a world of its own.

The sound of absolute silence is no better for sleep than noise, according to researchers. Volunteers have awakened and begun hallucinating in the absence of all sound. You are just as likely to wake up if there is a sudden silence after a previously steady noise, such as when an air-conditioner or radio turns off.

NOTE: Any sound over 70 decibels begins to activate your nervous system; 120 decibels marks the normal pain threshold.

Traffic on a relatively quiet city street	70–72 decibels
Sports car or truck	90 decibels
Vacuum cleaner	81 decibels
Loud power mower	107 decibels
Jet plane on takeoff	150 decibels

Lie down in darkness

Your body is extraordinarily sensitive to light. Even with your eyes closed, you can tell if it's midnight or midday. Your internal biological clock relies on light as one of its strongest time cues. Perhaps this is why it may be difficult for you to sleep when the light in the room is signaling you to wake up.

Heavy draperies or a special light-blocking shade can keep your room dark. Eye-shades may help if you are particularly sensitive to light or if you have to sleep during the day because of your schedule; however, be careful not to wear them too tightly. If you dislike the feeling of utter blackness, you can buy eyeshades with tiny pinholes to let muted light in. If you are more troubled by darkness than light, a small nightlight or a clock with an illuminated dial may be comforting and useful.

Mind over mattress

Samuel Clemens once recounted the story of a particularly difficult time he had falling asleep in a room with all the windows shut. After much tossing and muttering, he became impatient, picked up his shoe, and heaved it toward the window. At the sound of tinkling glass, he sighed with relief and promptly fell asleep. The next morning, he discovered that the windowpane was intact; he had sent his shoe flying into a glass-enclosed bookcase.

Benjamin Franklin also needed fresh air in order to sleep well. One night he was sharing a room with a man who insisted on keeping the shuttered windows closed. After considerable debate, Franklin won his point and triumphantly opened the shutters. The next morning, after a good night's sleep, he discovered that he had flung open the door to a small closet.

These anecdotes reveal more than the dubious merits of sleeping with a window open. They show how great a role your mind plays in your body's rest. If you *feel* there is something amiss in your sleep setting—if you think it is too hot, cold, noisy, bright, or stuffy—you will not rest well. This is why you should give special attention to the place in which you sleep. It is not important how your bedroom may look to others or whether it's precisely as cool, dark, and quiet as is recommended for most people. Make it right for *you*, so that it is a room that will comfort and cradle you through the nights of your life.

CHAPTER 7

Side-by-Side: Sleeping Together

S leeping together is the ultimate intimacy. In our society, the phrase "sleeping together" has become a euphemism for sexual intercourse. But even sexual partners may resist sharing a bed through the night. For them, sleep is more private and more vulnerable than sex.

Sleep and sex have more in common than the fact that both occur most often in bed. According to recent studies, sexuality both reflects and affects your nightly sleep. You will sleep differently if you sleep alone, together, or around.

Men and women may be guaranteed equality under the law by day, but they are not equal by night. Each sex is prone to different sleep problems, and each sex responds to sleep difficulties in characteristically different ways. Sexual differences continue to be apparent in the sleep patterns of couples who've shared the same bed for decades; these are observable even in dreams. Some couples find that sleep incompatibility is more of a problem than any daytime difficulty. One partner's sleep disorder, if not recognized and treated, can lead to sexual problems and feelings of rejection, resentment, or anger.

A couple spends more time sleeping together than in any daytime activity. Understanding what happens in bed—and why—may open both partners' eyes to another dimension of sexuality and intimacy.

How the sexes sleep

Biology alone does not determine the destiny of your nights. Your age and your health have more effect than your sex on how much sleep you need. Both men and women follow the same patterns of NREM and REM sleep in the night. However, men start spending less time in deep Stage 4 sleep in their thirties, while Stage 4 time does not decrease in women until they are in their fifties. Elderly adults of both sexes have less deep sleep than they did earlier in life.

A recent Gallup poll on sleeping habits found that more women than men say they actually sleep eight or more hours a night, and women are more likely to regard eight hours of sleep per night as ideal. Although more women slept longer, proportionately fewer men than women reported sleep difficulties. The greatest differences between men and women in this study was the frequency of sleep disturbances caused by nocturnal headaches (which affected 6.6 percent of the men and 16.5 percent of the women), a partner's restlessness or snoring (6.9 percent men and 18.1 percent women), and sleeping somewhere other than in one's regular bed (8.8 percent men and 13.3 percent women).

Single people reported more sleep difficulties than married ones, and a larger percentage of the unmarried respondents traced their problems to thinking over problems in bed or an inability to relax. The divorced and separated individuals went to bed later than the married ones and retired at different times from night to night.

Working women slept more like working men than like women who did not have careers outside their homes, spending fewer than eight hours in bed each night. Those who worked full-time slept less than women working part-time. However, they were less likely to report sleep problems than women with part-time jobs, who reported more sleep disruptions caused by headaches or muscle and joint aches. The widowed, divorced, and separated respondents had more sleep problems and generally discussed them with physicians, although women were more likely to seek such help than men. As men and women got older, the percentage of them who consulted their doctors about sleep problems increased.

Which is the weaker sex by night?

Women are twice as likely to complain about sleeplessness, to seek medical help for their sleep problems, and to take sleeping pills. However, men may have just as many—if not more—problems in bed. Not all sleep disorders discriminate between the sexes, but some definitely do.

Men actually are more vulnerable than women in the night. The overwhelming majority of the victims of apnea, a potentially lethal breathing disorder, are males. The various types of sleep apnea (see pages 192 and 227 for full descriptions) can lead to serious problems during the day as well as during the night, including extreme daytime sleepiness, inability to concentrate, irritability, and impotence. In one study, several men with sleep apnea traced their marital difficulties to their symptoms. Some were so tired because of their inability to sleep through the night that they fell asleep while making love with their wives. One man, estranged from his wife, was successfully treated for obstructive sleep apnea and was reconciled with her afterwards. Narcolepsy, another sleep problem characterized by irresistible daytime weariness, can lead to similar sexual and marital difficulties. The medications used to treat this illness (see page 222) also may cause impotence.

Men, who are more likely to develop heart diseases, may be more susceptible to nighttime irregularities in their heartbeats. Stanford University sleep researchers reported cases of "asystole" (no heart contractions) occurring periodically in the sleep of young men who showed no daytime signs of heart ailments. In some, the danger was so great that cardiac pacemakers were implanted.

Even as children, boys seem to have more problems during the night. Bed-wetting is more common in boys than girls and remains a problem longer. Boys may be more likely to take to their feet and become sleepwalkers than girls, and they may be more troubled by night terrors, the mysterious attacks of horror that occur during very deep sleep. One of the rarest sleep disorders is the Kleine-Levin syndrome which strikes adolescent males. Its victims seem to lose control of various appetites and periodically gorge themselves on food, become so sexually uninhibited that they may exhibit themselves in public, or sleep for inordinate amounts of time. Researchers suspect that this syndrome may be caused by hyperactivity in the brain, for the young men tend to be abnormally shy and withdrawn except during their binge periods (see page 233 for more information on this problem).

As adults, men tend to snore more frequently—and loudly—than women. They are more likely to suffer from REM-interruption insomnia (see page 211) and wake up during most of their nightly REM periods. Some researchers speculate that this may be their way of avoiding traumatic dreams. There also may be a preponderance of male victims of another, rarer problem—sleep drunkenness; these sleepers are unable to make the complete transition from sleep to wakefulness (see page 217).

One sleep problem that is uniquely and universally male is waking up because of painful erections. Victims usually have no sexual problems during the day, and researchers theorize that the intense pain accompanying their normal nighttime erections may be caused by a disorder of the sleep-controlling mechanisms of the brain (see page 248).

The sleep problems that plague women are those linked with their reproductive cycles. Adolescent girls may become extremely drowsy before and during their menstrual cycles. Excessive daytime tiredness can be one of the first signals of pregnancy. A mother-to-be, sleeping for two, usually adds two hours to her total sleep time through much of her pregnancy. However, she is likely to have more problems sleeping through the night in the final months before delivery (see page 249). The after-effects of the enormous hormonal changes of pregnancy and delivery can linger for months. Coupled with the demands of a newborn infant, it can be difficult for the new mother to sleep long or deeply enough to feel energetic through the day. Throughout her life, a woman's estrogen-progesterone balance is crucial to the way she feels. Her deep sleep typically declines after menopause, another time of hormonal upheaval.

Women may develop certain sleep disorders because of psychological rather than physiological reasons. The incidence of depression is significantly higher in women than in men, and sleep problems are generally one of the characteristic symptoms of this disorder (see page 214). Women also report more recurring dreams and nightmares. Since women are more likely to resort to the use of sleeping pills, their sleep problems may be compounded by dependence on these drugs (see page 185).

How the sexes dream

A man and a woman snuggling between the sheets may share the same bed, house, name, and lifestyle; yet they are worlds apart in their dreams. As researchers have shown, dreams in adulthood are as individual as fingerprints. And men and women continue to be as different by night as they are by day.

According to dream researcher, Milton Kramer, M.D., men's dreams tend to be more active and more friendly, yet they are more likely to include a fight scene. Other men that appear in a dream are likely to be antagonists. Men also dream more often of appearing naked in public. In recalling their dreams, men use nouns and describe things rather than people. And they dream about finding money more often than women do.

Women's dreams seem to reflect both biology and social conditioning. In 1939 Therese Benedek, the "foremother" of dream and gender studies, suggested that the sexual content of women's dreams is related to hormonal changes in the menstrual cycle. However, little research has been done to support this premise. Women do report dreams unlike men's in many ways. Women dream more often of being endangered or pursued, and their dreams take place in indoor rather than outdoor settings, usually with brightly colored decor and animated conversation. They generally use words of feeling and emotion to describe their dreams. The stereotypes of waking life persist in women's dreams. While both men and women dream of violation, men who feel exploited or abused dream of assault or robbery; women may express this feeling in a dream of being raped. According to psychologists, such rape dreams do not express an unconscious desire for sexual violence but are a parody of normal sexual relations. They may reflect a woman's anxiety and resentment about conventional relationships with men.

As women become more liberated, so do their dreams. More women are assuming so-called masculine roles in their dreams. Dream researcher Robert Van deCastle of the University of Virginia has reported that more women now identify people in their dreams by occupation, while once only men did so. The women in their dreams are more assertive and even physically aggressive. Rather than dreaming of courtship and weddings, today's women dream of vivid bedroom encounters, often extramarital ones. While women's sexual dreams once were quite prim and proper, limited to hugs and kisses, they now include scenes of passionate lovemaking, ending in orgasm. Even women who might be classified as "unliberated" by day are venturing into new territory by night.

Men and women consciously react differently to sexual dreams, particularly when a person of the same sex is in the dream. The women in one study dreamed equally about men and women in a sexual context and were not upset by the content of these dreams. The men hesitated to report sexual dreams about other men, as if fearful of an implication of homosexuality. When medical students were asked to report their dreams, they carefully "edited out" any such references in talking with faculty members. However, they did report them to researchers who had no relation to their academic work.

After studying the dream reports of 1,000 patients, one California psychologist concluded that women not only dream more about feelings but are more likely to have dream memories and feelings linger during the day. Women's daydreams are also unlike men's. In a major investigation of daydreams, researchers found that women show more curiosity about people than things, while men show equal curiosity about both. Males had significantly more daydreams about failing and guilt and more sexual daydreams than women, except for the ages from thirty-one to thirty-four, when women and men had equal numbers of sexual fantasies. However, women at all ages daydreamed more and with greater intensity than men.

Several studies have shown that women have more nightmares than men. Some suggest that poor women are most haunted by bad dreams; others suggest that the incidence of nightmares increases with age and that after age fifty they occur equally in men and women. Both sexes report repetitive dreams, usually unpleasant, but women seem more likely to experience recurring themes in their dreams. Sometimes "bad" dreams as well as good serve a beneficial purpose. In one Florida study of seventy women during their first pregnancies, many dreamed about their forthcoming deliveries, often visualizing great problems and deformed infants. The women who had these anxious dreams about delivery actually had shorter and easier labors than those who didn't. It could be that they gained control of their natural anxiety by dreaming.

Sleep and sexuality: what one says about the other

For a teenage boy, one of the typical signs of approaching sexual maturity occurs during sleep: a nocturnal orgasm or "wet" dream. The incidence of such dreams varies from 28 to 80 percent in various age groups, and they are particularly common in adolescence. But nighttime erections begin much earlier and have been observed in infants only days old. At first, researchers thought that males experience erections as they sleep because they are having sexual dreams. However, when the men were deprived of REM sleep, erections persisted in other sleep periods, appearing at the very time when REM might ordinarily appear. Although sexual dreams may not be the reason for nocturnal erections, they do affect them. Erections that occur during provocative dreams are larger and firmer than others. Some scientists believe that an erection may actually be the cue for a sexual dream. In other words, the brain may receive signals of sexual arousal and weave that response into an erotic dream (see page 49).

Nighttime erections are so common during sleep that their absence is an important sign of impaired sexual health. Sleep specialist Ismet Karacan, M.D., of Baylor University became intrigued by the possibility that monitoring nightly erections—or nocturnal penile tumescence—might be a means of determining the causes of impotence. In the past, impotence was diagnosed primarily on the basis of the patient's complaint. If no physical abnormality could be detected, doctors concluded the problem was psychological, a determination they made in 90 to 95 percent of all cases. Treatment was based on the premise that the key to the problem lay in the man's mind rather than his body. When Karacan and his colleagues began monitoring nocturnal tumescence, they came up with surprising findings: 60 percent of the impotent men had no nighttime erections, indicating that there was a physical cause for their problem. Because there was no objective and precise method of diagnosing impotence, physicians had overestimated psychological problems in impotent men. "As a result many men have not gotten the right treatment for their problem," says Karacan. "Surgeons are willing to implant prosthetic devices in cases of organic (physical) impotence so the man can resume sexual activity. In psychological impotence, they're reluctant to do so, and the emphasis is on psychotherapy."

Impotence is not uncommon. Virtually all men experience occasional problems in obtaining or maintaining an erection, particularly after age forty. Among the possible physical causes for chronic impotence are: diabetes, multiple sclerosis, kidney disease, paralysis of the lower body, and certain heart and blood vessel abnormalities. Medications for a wide range of physical ailments also can lead to impotence.

Scientists have suggested that there may be a female counterpart to nocturnal penile tumescence, possibly cyclic arousal of the clitoris during sleep or periodic lubrication of the vagina. However, little research has been done on the use of sleep studies as a diagnostic tool for female sexual dysfunction. Technology has not yet been developed to monitor the subtler signs of women's sexual response, and there are many ethical considerations that have discouraged such research.

Sex and sleep: what one does for the other

The couple gets in bed, embraces passionately, the movie camera delicately turns away, and when we next see the lovers, they are sleeping in each other's arms. Like many movie fantasies, this one doesn't necessarily hold true in real life.

Sex has been shown to induce sleep—in animals. A sexually aroused cat for example, cannot sleep unless it finds a mate; afterward, it settles into peaceful rest. Rabbits typically fall into REM sleep after coitus. Some biologists have suggested that sleep after sex may enhance the chances for conception. Perhaps this is one reason rabbits are so prolific.

What about the human animal? Will you sleep better after sex? This depends on whether you're male or female. For reasons as unfathomable as sexuality itself, sex has different effects on the way the sexes sleep. After intercourse, a man is more likely to fall asleep, and his sleep stages are unchanged. A woman, less likely to drift into sleep after sex, will get less deep NREM sleep and spend more of the night in REM sleep and the lighter NREM stages.

This difference between men and women may be partly a matter of sexual satisfaction. After his climax, a man may feel so relaxed that he falls asleep quickly and easily. But if the woman has not had an orgasm, she may feel physically restless and frustrated. Baylor University's sleep clinic has reported a remarkably high correlation between sexual and sleep problems in women. Sixty to 70 percent of the women who complained of insomnia also reported sexual frustration. Could sexual dysfunction be the cause of their disturbed sleep? Certainly, anyone who feels angry, disappointed, or sad is not going to fall asleep as quickly as one who is content. But the problem may be much more complex; even after orgasm, women tend to get less deep NREM sleep. It may be that sex leads to a much briefer relaxation period, perhaps just a few minutes long, in women.

There actually is little objective proof that sex helps men sleep better. In one experiment, a group of male volunteers abstained from sex for ten days while their sleep patterns were recorded in a laboratory. At the end of the period, each had sexual intercourse and then returned to the lab to sleep. Although the men *said* that they slept better and felt more refreshed and relaxed, the sleep recordings showed no difference in their sleep patterns. Of course, sleep monitors cannot measure subjective feelings, and sexual satisfaction may have effects too subtle to be picked up in recordings of brain waves or heart rate.

Sex can be a powerful experience—and for this reason it may *not* be a good sleep inducer. If it evokes feelings of anxiety, tension, or frustration in a couple, it may well lead to a bad night. If sex becomes a routine act performed by two weary bedmates as a matter of habit, it loses its zest and meaning. Tired lovers are poor lovers, and for many people, sex is more enjoyable when they're more alert, energetic, and responsive.

In animal experiments, sleep researchers found another unexpected relation between sex and sleep. When they deprived cats of REM sleep, the animals became much more sexually aggressive. Could the lack of vivid dreams somehow influence the factors that determine sexual appetite? No one knows for sure. But there is evidence for some link between sleep and sexual control in humans with the Kleine-Levin syndrome (see page 233).

Two for the bed

A shared bed may be all that a sleeping couple has in common through the night. Scientists recorded the sleep patterns of two couples over the course of a week as they slept together according to their regular schedule, slept separately on the same schedule, and slept together without a schedule. They found that each individual's sleep cycles remained independent of the other's. Their conclusion was that a sleeping couple is really more separate than together.

Other studies have shown that women sleep more poorly than their bedmates. Typically, deep NREM sleep is briefer for women than for men sharing the same bed. And the men may be the reason why. They are more likely to snore than the women, and their nightly serenades may awaken the women from even the deepest sleep. Men are also more prone to disorders that involve major body movements, and their flailing limbs may rouse the women and force them to retreat. Or it may be a case of one mate pulling weight on the other. Each time the man rolls over, his movement may jar the women, perhaps not to the point of waking her, but she may go into a lighter sleep stage. If there's a difference of more than fifty pounds in weight, the woman may find herself sliding into a "trough" in the mattress, which forms as her bedmate shifts his weight. One sleep researcher has noted that each time one person in a double bed moves, the other moves within twenty seconds.

But there is one well-documented exception to this rule. In photographing sleeping couples at fifteen-minute intervals throughout the night, a researcher found that the one couple who slept "in tandem," with their body positions and sleep cycles tightly synchronized through two REM-NREM cycles, had spent a prolonged period of time making love before falling asleep. This experience, presumably satisfying to both partners, may have brought them together in sleep.

One problem with trying to determine whether individuals sleep better in pairs is that sleep monitoring equipment cannot pick up intangibles, like feelings of security and intimacy when sleeping together. However, sleep recordings do show disrupted sleep patterns in couples who take to separate beds, for whatever reason, after becoming accustomed to sharing a bed. When bedmates slept separately in a sleep laboratory, for instance, both showed an increase in REM and a decrease in deep NREM sleep. And separated, divorced, and bereaved people are much more likely to have sleep problems. It also seems more than coincidental that unmarried people who sleep alone or do not have a regular bed partner report more sleep difficulties than married couples.

The way two people sleep together may change drastically over time, and the sleep positions that two people choose at the start of the night may reflect their relationship through the day. According to psychiatrist Samuel Dunkell, new lovers may sleep nestled together like spoons, in semifetal positions, one partner tucked into the contours of the other partner's body. This coziness provides each partner with reassurance by offering maximum physical intimacy. After five years or so, the partners begin to drift apart, and there is a widening gulf between their bodies when they choose the "spoon position." They may totally shift positions so that they are sleeping back to back, with only their feet touching. Ultimately they may return to the favored positions of their youth. This physical retreat does not necessarily represent an emotional rift, says Dunkell, who feels it may be a testimony to the mutual security the couple has achieved. However, if once-cuddly partners suddenly move to opposite ends of the bed, this can be a sign that something is amiss.

Coping with problems in bed

The first night you spend with someone is like a first date in darkness: you are on your best sleep behavior. Each of you may agree to your partner's preferences about turning the light off or leaving it on, opening the window or turning up the thermostat. You may give up "your" side of the bed or forsake your customary sleep position in order to hold or be held by your new bedmate. The night may be romantic, but for many reasons, you aren't likely to sleep well.

Even when you are no longer strangers in the night, you may find that two do not sleep as easily as one. You may have incompatible sleep rituals or styles. What if your bed partner does yoga in the nude before bed while you like to fling open the window and snuggle under the covers with cookies and milk? What if one person likes music and the other prefers white noise (see page 79)? What if the mattress seems hard to one person and soft to the other? How many blankets are enough? Should the cat be allowed its usual place at the foot of the bed? What about your allergies? At least the fairytale princess who couldn't sleep because of a pea dozens of mattresses beneath her didn't have a mate insisting the problem was all in her head, so would she please turn over and go to sleep.

These may sound like trivial issues, but when a couple starts losing sleep over them, they become very serious. Your daily lives together can show the strain of your nighttime discord. Is it worth turning the bed into a battleground? In these situations, compromises are desirable and are usually possible. If one person's night-light is a nuisance to the other person, buy a pair of eyeshades. If one is cold while the other is hot, get an electric blanket with separate settings for each sleeper. If one thinks the mattress is too hard and the other disagrees, try two separate mattresses joined together in a common frame. If one person complains of being shoved around each time the other moves, consider a bigger bed. If no bed is big enough to accommodate all your sleep differences, you may want to opt for twin beds. It is better to be apart at night than let your nightly difficulties push you apart by day.

A much more complicated issue is how to cope if one partner has a sleep disorder. The individual who is lying in bed, wide-eyed and worried about falling asleep, may not gaze with fondness at the person a few inches away who fell asleep the minute the lights went out. And the good sleeper may run out of patience when awakened by the kicks of a mate with nocturnal myoclonus (see page 199), or the snores of someone with obstructive sleep apnea (see page 223), or the fussing of someone who wakes up frequently through the night.

These may be problems the two of you cannot work out alone. Talk the matter over and encourage your sleepless mate to seek proper help. Be wary of suggesting sleeping pills; you may discover that the problem becomes worse because of reliance on medications for sleep (see page 185). If a sleep ritual or relaxation technique may help, join your partner; you may feel better as well. If the problem is triggered by daytime stress, you both should try to recognize what is causing the pressure and what can be done about it.

Sometimes the daytime symptoms of a sleep problem are the most perplexing to a spouse. How do you respond if your mate suddenly collapses because of a narcoleptic sleep attack (see page 222)? How do you remain tolerant when your partner falls asleep while you are making love? What if the medications prescribed for a particular sleep problem cause sexual difficulties? These issues are real and troubling, and they cannot be overcome unless they are recognized. In some cases, you may want to seek supportive help in maintaining your part of the relationship. And remember that the better you understand your partner's sleep disorder, the better you'll be able to cope with it.

Few relationships that thrive only in bed or only away from the bed endure for very long. When two people share a bed, they share an important, intimate part of each other's life. The person you sleep with is a person you trust. The more nights you spend together, the closer you become. In the darkness of night, you can strengthen the bonds that keep you together during the day.

◆　　◆　　◆

Rate Your Mate's Sleeping Habits

Men and women sleep differently at night. How well do you know how the opposite sex sleeps? The following quiz, adapted from material from the Better Sleep Council, may test your nocturnal knowledge:

1 ◆ *A plane flies low over your house. Who is more likely to wake up?*
   (a) the man (b) the woman
2 ◆ *Who dreams in more vivid colors?*
   (a) the man (b) the woman
3 ◆ *Who is more apt to be disturbed when the bedmate changes positions?*
   (a) the man (b) the woman
4 ◆ *Who usually needs more sleep?*
   (a) the man (b) the woman
5 ◆ *The baby cries. Who is more likely to wake up?*
   (a) the man (b) the woman
6 ◆ *Who is more likely to daydream about failure and guilt?*
   (a) the man (b) the woman
7 ◆ *Who is more likely to have nightmares?*
   (a) the man (b) the woman
8 ◆ *When a man and woman sleep together, who sleeps more deeply?*
   (a) the man (b) the woman

Answers:
1 ◆ b, the woman. Women are more likely to awaken to airplane noises than men; older people also are more sensitive than younger people.
2 ◆ b, the woman. After studying the dreams of 1,000 patients over a three-year period, a University of California psychologist found that women reported significantly more color in their dreams.
3 ◆ b, the woman. Because she's lighter, she'll be disturbed when her bed partner shifts position. A difference of fifty pounds or more can create a "trough" in the bed into which the lighter person may roll.
4 ◆ Both the man and the woman. The amount of sleep needed varies with metabolism, health, and emotional well-being, not sex.

5 ◆ b, the woman. *In most instances the woman is the primary care giver to a child and responds more quickly to its cries. If the husband is sharing equal responsibility, he would be just as likely to wake up.*

6 ◆ a, the man. *Men also have more sexual daydreams than women, except for the age period between thirty-one and thirty-four, when both sexes daydream equally about sex.*

7 ◆ b, the woman. *Women report more nightmares up to the age of fifty, after which both sexes seem to experience them equally.*

8 ◆ a, the man. *Women seem to sleep less deeply for several reasons, including disruptions when their mates change sleep positions or snore.*

This information provided courtesy of the Better Sleep Council, P.O. Box 275, Burtonsville, MD. 20730.

◆   ◆   ◆

CHAPTER 8

Sleep Styles and Rituals:
Now I Lay Me Down to Sleep

B y day you may crave individuality. You cultivate an image, a look, a lifestyle that distinguishes you from others. But by night you want to be just like the people around you: sound asleep. Vladimir Nabokov once described sleep as "the most moronic fraternity in the world, with the heaviest dues and the crudest rituals." Yet it's a fraternity everyone wants to join.

There are rules in this anything-but-elite club, and there are exceptions to each one. There is no such thing as an "ideal" or "typical" sleeper, sleep duration, or presleep ritual. You may go to bed at night like everyone else, but you do so with a style all your own.

You may think you are most mysterious at night, when you lie in silence and darkness, but you're far from anonymous. Your sleep needs, preferences, rituals, positions, what you wear—or don't wear—are all distinctively yours. Recognizing individual differences is important in determining whether a person's nightlife is marred by a sleep problem or simply marked by an unusual sleep pattern. Understanding what happens before and after you get into bed also may help you to ease your transition from day into night and to recognize how what you do by day affects how you sleep by night.

How much sleep do you need?

Some researchers say the Romans partitioned the day into thirds and allotted one-third for sleep. Others credit the twelfth-century philosopher Maimonides with declaring that we should spend 8 of every 24 hours asleep. Whoever deserves the credit also should get some blame. However, 8 hours of sleep is *not* a reasonable or desirable goal for everyone; the natural, normal range of sleep time in humans is 5 to 10 hours. Approximately one person in one hundred may be able to get by with just 5 hours; another 1 percent will need twice as much sleep. The world-wide average for daily sleep time is 7½ hours, but there are dramatic exceptions. A Spanish man allegedly slept less than 1 hour a day; an Australian slept for 3 hours; an English woman slept for 1 or 2 hours. What is most remarkable about these short sleepers is not just how little they sleep but how efficiently they rest. Sleep recordings have shown that short sleepers spend just as much time as the average person in the deep, restorative stages of NREM sleep and the same proportion of their sleep time in REM sleep. What they do without are the "filler" stages of light NREM sleep through the night.

Sleep needs seem to be part of genetic programming, along with hair color, height, and skin tone. Just as you may be tall, short, or average in height, you might sleep for long, short, or average periods of time. Your sleep needs change during your lifetime, according to your age, metabolism, health, physical activity, job demands, and emotional state. You may sleep less in your twenties than you did as a teenager. Life situations have a significant impact on how much sleep you need and get. A pregnant woman may add an hour to her daily sleep. Generally, people sleep more when worried or under stress; sleep may actually help restore and strengthen you in times of crisis. Your body may signal you to go to bed when you are coming down with a cold or flu; sleep is also extended—and essential—in recovery from serious injury or illness. When all is going well, you usually sleep less but feel more energetic.

It is easy to figure out how much sleep you need. One way is to get up at the same time every morning, regardless of when you go to bed. Is it difficult for you to get up after only six hours of rest? Do you feel more energetic after seven hours? Let your body teach you how much sleep suits you best. Another method is to keep track of how much you sleep on weekends, when you can sleep as late and as long as you'd want. If you feel noticeably better when you extend your sleep time on Saturday and Sunday, this may be a sign that you are not getting enough sleep during the week. Remember, though, that too much sleep can make you feel sleepy!

Can you get by on less sleep?

Everyone gets too little sleep once in a while. You may stay up late cramming for a test or partying. You may cut down on sleep time in order to meet a deadline, work on a special project, or care for a sick child. You may feel less than terrific in the meantime, but you manage to keep your eyes open. The reason for this is motivation. If you have enough reason to stay awake, you'll be less interested in getting more sleep. But how long can you keep sacrificing your sleep time? Is it possible to get by on less sleep for extended periods of time? The answer isn't clear, but it does seem that you can sleep a little less (probably a maximum of forty-five to sixty minutes less each night) and continue to function well.

In one experiment, sleep researchers asked three couples—who usually slept 8 hours a night—and a fourth couple—who slept 6½ hours—to cut down on their sleep by 30 minutes a night every 2 weeks until they were sleeping 6 hours a night. Then they were told to cut their sleep by 30 minutes at 3-week intervals. The couples succeeded: one couple reduced their sleep time to 4½ hours; two couples, to 5 hours; one couple to 5½ hours. The partners were then told to sleep as much as they wanted to. A year later the researchers found that six of the eight partners were still sleeping 1 to 2½ hours less each night than they had when the experiment began, with no complaints about daytime or nighttime problems.

The volunteers in this experiment were young—undergraduate or graduate students between the ages of twenty-one and twenty-eight. Their age may have made it easier for them to alter their sleep habits, although the gradual reduction may have been the key to success. If you genuinely want to sleep less, either temporarily or permanently, don't suddenly reduce your sleep by two hours. If you slowly cut back your sleep time, you may be able to gain up to an extra hour a day.

Nightcaps and midnight snacks

The world's oldest and most popular sleep aid is a nip of alcohol. As long as it's just a nip, it works. A glass of wine or a bit of brandy will shorten the time until you fall asleep, but overindulgence will disrupt your sleep patterns in the second half of the night. You may wake up before dawn, hung over and unable to get back to sleep (see page 219).

Other sleep-inducing nightcaps are nonalcoholic. Herbal teas have been used for centuries, particularly those made of chamomile, one of the oldest sedatives. A favorite Chinese drink is ginseng and dried orange juice mixed with honey. Others mix cider vinegar and honey. And you can always drink a glass of warm milk. Lately there has been much enthusiasm over the discovery that L-tryptophan, an amino acid found in milk and other dairy products, may be nature's own sleeping pill. Scientists say that one to ten grams of this natural substance may help you fall asleep faster (see page 148). However, there is far too little tryptophan in a single glass of milk to have any substantial effect. One small study several years ago did show that malted milk was stronger and more effective than a placebo (an inactive substance) in shortening sleep latencies, although this has not been verified.

Some cultures prefer to eat rather than drink at bedtime: the English recommend chewing an apple slowly before going to bed; Pueblo Indians suggest mushrooms; the Burmese eat a pollen cake. Some nutritionists say that what you eat earlier in the day also affects your sleep. In addition to substances containing caffeine, they propose that two possible culprits in sleep problems are sugar and salt, two of the most common ingredients in the American diet. Vitamin deficiencies and poor eating habits are also likely to disrupt sleep.

In laboratory experiments, the less food that rats were given, the less they slept. After six to eleven days of food deprivation, they seemed to stop sleeping, perhaps because of their survival instincts—hunger may keep them awake so they can hunt for food. The relationship between food and sleep does not seem so clear-cut in humans. However, one study suggests that people who recently lost weight complained more about poor sleep and frequent awakenings than those who gained weight or stayed at the same weight. Yet some poor sleepers seem particularly tempted to snack before bed or when they awaken in the night. It may be that food is a comfort to them, especially if they feel anxious about their sleep or dreams.

If you do wake up hungry in the night, keep in mind that the morning weigh-in will reflect calories eaten in the dark as well as in the day. Keep low-calorie snacks, such as celery, apples, skim milk, and juices, available. If you reward yourself for waking up in the night by finishing the lemon meringue pie, you are giving yourself a reason to wake up again the next night. You might end up not only weary but fat.

Sleep security

Even wolf packs have young males who watch while the others sleep. Humans are no different than any other species in regard to sleep security: they cannot rest well unless they feel safe. If you lie awake in bed, particularly when your bed partner is away, you're sure to hear something go bump in the night. This is the nature of pipes and roofs and shutters. However, if you take some extra security precautions, you should be reassured about your safety. Here are some practical suggestions:

• Make sure there are locks on all the doors and windows. Install a burglar alarm system if you feel it's necessary or desirable.
• Buy a smoke detector, and make sure it's set loud enough to rouse you from sleep. Hold a fire drill so everyone knows what to do and how to get out of the house just in case.
• If you hop out of bed in the middle of the night to check the pilot light on the kitchen stove or the screen on the back door, make it part of your sleep ritual to do a thorough safety check before you go to sleep.
• Install an extension phone at your bedside. Write the numbers for emergency help, fire, and police on a label and put it on the phone.
• If the dark disturbs you, keep a night-light on and get a clock with a luminous dial.
• If you wear glasses, keep them in the same spot each night so you can reach them without fumbling.
• Try one of the sound-muffling sleep devices described on page 79.

What does all this have to do with sleep? These suggestions are the means to peace of mind—a prerequisite for a good night's sleep.

Sleep rituals: whatever happened to counting sheep?

There's a reason why so many people have counted so many sheep for so many years in order to get to sleep: It works. The reason, according to researchers, is that counting sheep distracts both halves of your brain with a soothing, repetitive activity. The left brain, which is involved in logical calculations, does the counting. The right brain, which produces visual images, conjures up the wooly coats and damp black eyes. Preoccupied with the sheep, skipping through your mind, you bore yourself to sleep.

If the thought of so much wool makes you itch, there are other exercises that use a similar strategy. For example, you might imagine that you are writing perfect numerals six feet high on an imaginary blackboard. Start at 100 and go backwards to 0.

Or you can tell yourself a pleasant story. Think of a beautiful natural scene, such as a beach or waterfall, complete with appropriate sound effects. Put yourself into this setting and describe what you are seeing and hearing. Pay special attention to details: the moon in the sky, the rushing water, the blue-green waves, the sea gulls.

You also might try talking to yourself—or rather talking yourself to sleep. Repeat the phrase, "I am going to sleep, I am going to sleep," in a quiet, even voice. Don't make any conscious effort to sleep, just listen to your own words. This type of autosuggestion is a form of self-hypnosis that is remarkably effective. You might want to combine it with some simple stretching exercises.

Most sleep rituals are rather mundane: a warm bath, light reading, listening to soft music, talking with a bedmate. Even the simple act of changing into pajamas and turning out the light is part of the routine that signals your body to prepare for sleep. You might not think you have a presleep ritual—until you get into bed one night with the sense that you have left something undone. That "something" might be brushing your teeth, or laying out tomorrow's clothes, or watching Johnny Carson. Whatever it is, it is your personal way of turning yourself off for the night.

So what if you sleep in the nude?

Sleeping nude may expose a lot of flesh, but it doesn't reveal any unusual psychological forces. In many countries, sleeping nude is a matter of cultural habit; in ours, it is a matter of personal preference.

An estimated 40 percent of adult women and 25 percent of men sleep naked. Nocturnal nudists don't seem more or less likely to develop sleep problems; and they keep warm and comfortable by adding an extra layer of blankets if necessary. However, if you suddenly strip for bed after years of wearing pajamas or a nightgown, you may feel less comfortable—and less able to sleep.

What do people wear to bed? Almost anything soft and loose, from underwear to football t-shirts to flannel pajamas to slinky gowns. You may find that the sexiest bed fashions, layered with lace and trimmed with feathers, are less than cozy in bed. When it comes to sleeping, choose the garments that feel best. You don't want to spend the night tugging at a too-tight waistband or sweating in a long-sleeved, buttoned-up nightshirt.

Sleep positions: night language of the body?

You may think you've "slept like a log" after a good night's rest, but if you actually did lie motionless through the night, you would wake up feeling like a felled tree. In a typical night you may move forty to seventy times as you sleep. Such shifts prevent the pooling of blood in your inert body, keep the oxygen and carbon dioxide exchange constant, and maintain muscle tone.

There may be a characteristic pattern to the way you move during the night and the positions you take, just as there is a distinctive style to your gestures and postures during the day. Sleep studies suggest that sleep movements tend to be highly individual. A sleeper has a repertoire of favorite positions, including some that are mirror images of each other and are alternately assumed through the night.

Could the positions you choose by night express your feelings from the day? Sleep researchers are dubious. The reasons for choosing a sleep position may have much more to do with physiology than psychology. One sleep researcher begins his general lectures with two slides: one of his daughter as a little girl, fast asleep with her head on the pillow and her rump up in the air; the other of a polar bear in the same sleep position. Some unusual sleep positions or movements can be a sign of sleep problems. Repeated leg jerks in the night are characteristics of victims of nocturnal myoclonus (page 199). Sleepers with breathing disorders (see sections on apnea, pages 192 and 227) may flail about wildly in the night and collapse propped up against a wall or leaning against the bed. Young children may rock themselves to sleep; occasionally their movements seem violent as they bang their heads into their pillow or mattress (see page 263). Perhaps the most mysterious movements of all are those of sleepwalkers, who may climb stairs, open doors, or even drive a car (see page 200).

Most of us are far more restrained as we sleep, but external factors do influence our nightly pantomime. One study indicated that your mattress affects your movements. Volunteers who slept on a hard carpet-covered board moved the most; those sleeping on a featherbed also moved often. The volunteers sleeping on a standard innerspring mattress had the lowest movement rate.

Other possible influences on sleep movement include caffeine and heavy meals (both increased sleep movements) and alcohol (which decreased motion early in the night but increased movements during the latter half). If the sleep of intoxicated persons doesn't lighten over the course of the night, they will wake up feeling stiff and achy—as well as hung over. Body weight may also make a difference in movement. Thin people may move more on a hard mattress because they lack natural cushioning. On the other hand, sleepers who are heavy may sink so far down into a soft mattress that they find it difficult to move around easily.

The muscles of the limbs and torso are usually limp during REM sleep. But one night a sleep researcher observed his wife twitching her legs as she slept. After being awakened, she said that she had been dancing in her dreams. According to some dream researchers, a change in position during REM sleep may be a signal or even a trigger for a scene shift in a dream.

Could there be more to sleep positions than muscle movements or dream scenes? Psychiatrist Samuel Dunkell, who wrote a book called *Sleep Positions*, correlated his patients' daytime problems with their sleep postures. For example, an insecure person would curl up in a fetal position, almost as if the bed were a womb. An egotistical individual, supremely confident, would lie on his or her back, arms flung to either side and feet spread apart. Generally, the more bizarre the person's daytime behavior, the more bizarre the sleep position was. Some of Dunkell's patients twisted themselves into contortions that most of us would find impossible to mimic.

Studying your own sleep posture probably won't lead to new insights about yourself, but it can be amusing to look at the similarities between how you act by day and how you settle down for sleep once you get into bed. If you are meticulously organized all day, you might be just as fastidious about arranging sheets, blankets, and pillow before you sleep. If you are a "people" person and hate to be alone by day, you may feel most cozy curled up amid pillows or stuffed animals. If you are shy and inhibited during the day, you may be quiet and still by night as well.

There are practical reasons to be attentive to your sleep posture. If you sleep on your stomach, you may twist your neck into an unnatural, forward thrust, and your back won't get the support it needs. Sleeping on your back is better than lying face down, particularly if you put several pillows under your knees to prevent low back strain. A too-thick pillow also can bend you out of shape.

You can train yourself to take an ideal sleep position when you get into bed: Lie on your side, with spine straight, knees and elbows relaxed, limbs free of the body, shoulders and hips anchored. You can shift your hands and feet to whatever positions are comfortable for you.

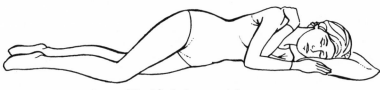

The ideal sleep position.

What your sleep time says about you

People who sleep much more or much less than average may have distinctive personality traits. Do they sleep differently because of their different views of the world? Or do they approach life differently because of their unusual sleep patterns? This is a chicken-and-egg question that no one has answered yet. But sleep researcher Dr. Ernest Hartmann of Tufts University has found an intriguing correlation between specific personality types and unusual sleepers. He believes that short sleepers—those who spend less than 5½ hours in bed—tend to be extroverted, efficient, ambitious people who work hard and feel fairly confident about themselves and satisfied with their lives. Long sleepers—who spend 9 hours or more in bed—tend to be introverted, anxious, insecure, and indecisive personalities, who worry more and ruminate over the day past and the day to come.

There is considerable disagreement about the validity of such psychological profiles. Other studies have found the opposite correlations; some experiments on sleep time have uncovered no personality differences at all. Researchers also differ in their conclusions about short and long sleepers. Is it better to be perky and ambitious and sleep less? Studies at San Jose State University indicate that short sleepers may also be "Type A" personalities who are at a higher risk of developing heart disease. Are long sleepers less capable by day? Not necessarily, since this category includes more nonconventional thinkers and creative people.

Australian scientists tried to learn more about personality by looking at the quality of sleep and sleep habits of 104 medical students. They found some proof for the old adage about early birds getting the worm. The early-rising students were better sleepers (73 percent said their sleep was very good), got better grades, and were conscientious and realistic about themselves. The students who got up an average of forty-two minutes later, both during the week and on weekends, were more likely to complain about their sleep, got poorer grades, and were rebellious and unrealistic about their capabilities and limitations.

The students' sleep problems were also revealing. Those who complained of difficulties falling asleep were almost always worriers, and their personality tests revealed that they had more anxiety and lower self-esteem than their peers. However, they had few physical symptoms. The students who woke up frequently in the night tended to repress their problems and had trouble admitting to any difficulties in their personal relationships. They also had a high incidence of physical complaints, such as weakness or dizziness.

Sleeping off the job

Does what you do for a living affect how you sleep at night? Absolutely. The effect is dramatic in some occupations. Truck drivers, pilots, doctors, nurses, sailors, soldiers, waitresses, entertainers, taxi drivers, air traffic controllers, train engineers, telephone operators—these are just a few of the people who may need to adjust their sleep time to their job schedules. The consequences of such change can be serious (see page 241).

Even if you work standard daytime hours, your job can have an impact on your nighttime sleep—whether you are an employer or an employee. Do you think that sales representatives and secretaries sleep better than their bosses? Once an executive has made it to the top, do you suppose he or she can relax and sleep an extra hour in the morning? Think again.

According to a recent survey of the presidents and chairpersons of the nation's Fortune 500 companies, executives slept less but reported fewer sleep problems than their employees. While the national average sleep time is 7½ hours, 46 percent of the business leaders slept an hour less. Only 36 percent slept more than 7 hours; 15 percent were in bed for 5 to 6 hours; two percent slept only 4 to 5 hours.

Such short nights seemed to be a matter of personal preference rather than an inability to sleep. Almost half—46 percent—said they had no difficulty falling asleep; another 47 percent said they had problems only occasionally. While 37 percent usually woke up during the night, 55 percent did so only some of the time and 7 percent never recalled awakening before dawn. Ninety percent of the executives did not take daytime naps.

What did these corporate leaders do when they couldn't sleep? Reading was their top choice (44 percent); much smaller percentages resorted to sleeping pills (16 percent), aspirin (15 percent), or a glass of warm milk (13 percent). Ten percent relaxed through sexual activity; 9 percent meditated; 8 percent had a drink; 5 percent exercised; 3 percent took a warm bath. They also did not worry too much about the consequences of a poor night's sleep, and more than half reported few negative effects the morning after.

Regardless of what you do, your satisfaction with your job may be as important to your sleep as the hours you work or how strenuous your daily duties are. If you are unhappy on the job, you might well have problems sleeping after work. If you are under financial pressure and have taken on extra work, you may be more tired than ever but have more problems sleeping. And if you are a full-time worker and a full-time homemaker, parent, and spouse— as 23 million American women are—you may not be able to sleep well at night because you spend the evening trying to catch up with household chores.

Naps: pajama-less sleep

A nap has been defined as "any rest episode up to twenty minutes in duration involving unconsciousness but not pajamas." Napping is a favorite human pastime. College students, whose schedules allow them to indulge in this habit, usually take at least one nap a week; in one study, 42 percent took five or more siestas a week. And the older you get, the more tempting the idea of an afternoon rest may be. In a study of people of different ages, those between forty and fifty years old took fewer than six naps over an eight-week period; those between fifty and sixty years old took slightly more than six; the sixty to seventy-year-olds took more than eleven naps; virtually all of those over eighty years old napped.

Many people are furtive nappers; others are candid. Winston Churchill, an advocate of catnapping, wrote, "Nature had not intended man to work from eight in the morning until midnight without the refreshment of blessed oblivion, which, even if it lasts only 20 minutes, is sufficient to renew all vital forces." John D. Rockefeller used to take an afternoon nap when he was in his forties; the older he got, the more he napped—until he regularly took five naps a day. Napoleon and Thomas Edison, notoriously short sleepers, napped during the day, as did General Douglas MacArthur and President John Kennedy.

Sleep experts believe that naps can interfere with sleep at night, even though they may be refreshing during the day. A morning nap, they found, tends to decrease REM periods the following night; you are also most likely to dream in the daytime if you nap before noon. An afternoon nap will be dreamless and will cut down on the time you spend in deep NREM sleep that night. Napping makes sleep less "efficient" so that you sleep less and less deeply, even if you spend more time in bed. Sometimes eliminating naps helps a person fall asleep more quickly and sleep longer through the night.

There seem to be differences in people who nap and those who do not—as well as differences among various nappers. A psychologist at the University of Pennsylvania classified nappers as either "replacement" nappers, who slept in the day to make up for sleep lost at night, or "appetitive" nappers, who rested during the day because they liked to, even when not feeling tired. In his study of 261 nappers, 78 percent napped to replace lost sleep. However, both types fell asleep within twelve minutes when they lay down to nap and both awoke

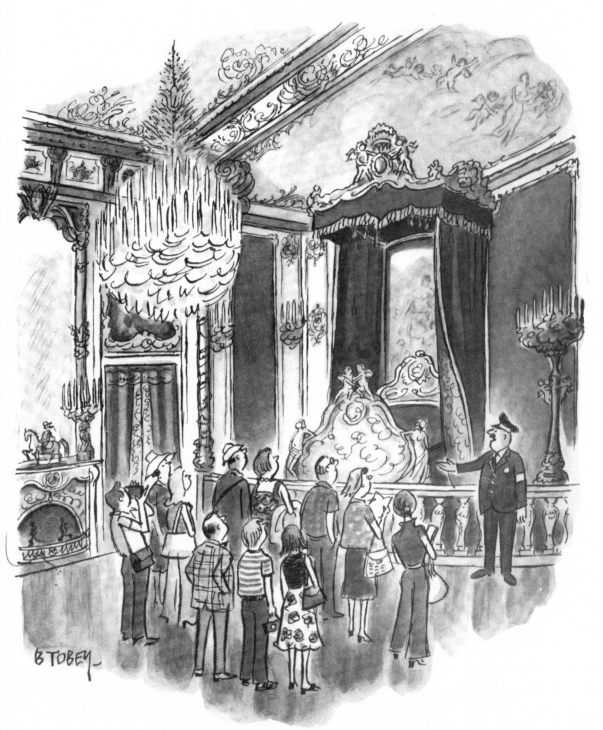

"His Royal Highness was a night person."

Drawing by B Tobey; © 1980 The *New Yorker* Magazine, Inc.

feeling refreshed. Nonnappers, by comparison, required twenty-six minutes to drift off during the day and awoke feeling less rested. At night the appetitive nappers spent more time in the lighter stages of sleep and moved frequently from one sleep stage to another. The replacement nappers had fewer sleep changes and more deep sleep. However, none of the nappers slept like nonnappers do.

The tendency to grow drowsy through the day may be the result of our fluctuating circadian rhythms (see "Sunrise, Sunset," page 15); napping may be something some people need more than others. If it is difficult for you to sleep at night, you will be better off staying awake during the day. However, for some people with flexible schedules, napping may be the answer to chronic sleep deprivation and daytime tiredness. In studies by Stanford University researcher Mary Carskadon, college students reported that they had more energy if they scheduled an afternoon nap. A physician in Louisiana prescribed naps for several hundred women who complained of feeling nervous and fatigued; about two-thirds reported that they felt better during the day and slept better at night.

It may not be the daytime sleep per se but "the pause that refreshes." There is no physiological explanation for why a few minutes of midday sleep should provide an extraordinary degree of restoration. It may well be that the relaxation of the muscles, the break in conscious thought processes, and the escape from anxiety are what actually refresh the catnapper.

If this is true, there may be alternatives to napping that can help you through the day without affecting your sleep at night. You might take a few minutes to practice a relaxation technique (see page 113). Or you could close your eyes and conjure up a soothing scene, complete with sound. Or you could take a series of long, deep breaths. Walk away from your work for a few moments; stretch; sigh; yawn; tense and relax your muscles. Within a few minutes, your body will shift toward the "up" part of its ninety-minute activity cycle and you will feel more energetic.

What not to do in bed

There are more appropriate hours in the day for many activities that will make you more aroused and far less sleepy. Here is a list of some of the activities *not* to do in bed:

1 ◆ Balance your checkbook

2 ◆ Discuss the household budget with your mate

3 ◆ Weigh yourself (you are heaviest at night so you will probably be discouraged)

4 ◆ Read a gory mystery

5 ◆ Mull over the possible consequences of nuclear war

6 ◆ Ponder what inflation will be like in the year 2000

7 ◆ Rerun a scene of embarrassment or failure from the preceding day

8 ◆ Think of all the things you should have said

9 ◆ Eat a pepperoni pizza or a burrito

10 ◆ Tell your spouse about your run-in with a highway patrol officer, another car, or a remarkably charming insurance broker

The time when you get into bed is the time to leave behind the cares of the day and enter another dimension of life. Recognizing your sleep style and accommodating your schedule and habits to your sleep needs will help you make this transition much more easily.

CHAPTER 9

Techniques to Help You Sleep Better

Y ou take care of yourself by day, and you can take charge of what happens to you at night. For the most part, you can do much more than any physician—or any pill—to help yourself sleep better. While some sleep disorders can be diagnosed and treated only by specialists trained in sleep medicine, you can tackle many common sleep problems on your own, without relying on sleeping pills. This chapter describes effective alternatives to pills that can help you help yourself in the night.

Relaxation techniques

"Relax," your friend or physician may say when you complain about your sleep problems. But relaxing is no simple matter, particularly if you are trying to become relaxed enough to sleep.

There are specific approaches to relaxation that, with practice and patience, can help you sleep. Researchers have not proved that one method is better than the others. All can work—if you master the techniques that help you induce a profound state of relaxation.

Some people can quickly learn these techniques on their own; others prefer to take classes with professional therapists. You may be able to get to sleep simply by performing a few basic exercises in bed, or you may prefer a systematic relaxation program. Whichever approach you choose, practice is essential. Cassette tapes, along with self-help guides, are available for many of the techniques.

One sign that the relaxation therapies are working is awareness of new and different sensations during the exercises, such as feelings of floating, warmth, or heaviness. Initially, these unfamiliar feelings may seem unsettling, even unpleasant. Some people may cry out or twitch or feel sudden anxiety; a trained teacher is prepared for such temporary problems.

Relaxation techniques work best for people with muscular tension who have problems falling asleep. Studies have shown that these approaches work better than a placebo in inducing sleep. And they may work on the mind as well as the body by providing the sleepless person with a new sense of control and self-confidence. Think of relaxation therapy as a new coping skill that will make you feel less helpless—and more sleepy.

Progressive muscle relaxation (PMR)

Progressive or deep muscle relaxation was developed in 1930 by Edmund Jacobson, M.D., and has been used in helping people with headaches, allergic reactions, and stress-related maladies. The basic exercise involves alternate tensing and relaxing of various muscle groups in the body. Attention is focused on a specific muscle group, such as the arm muscles: you tense them tightly and then release them. The tension-relaxation exercises become more effective each time you do them, so you become progressively more relaxed in less time. They also teach you to recognize what your body feels like when its muscles are very tense and very relaxed. Focusing your attention on this process becomes relaxing in itself.

The PMR exercises take time and practice, usually twenty to thirty minutes a session. You shouldn't try using this technique at bedtime until you have become proficient through daily practice. Here is a step-by-step guide:

1 ◆ Make sure your setting is comfortable. For daytime practice, use a quiet spot and easy chair. For nighttime, make yourself as comfortable as possible in bed.
2 ◆ When you're tensing your muscles, do so vigorously, but not so much that you develop a cramp. Hold the muscle in its tensed position for five to seven seconds; count 1001, 1002, 1003, and so on, to time the contraction. Relax for fifteen to twenty seconds.

3 ◆ Concentrate on what is happening. Feel the buildup of tension; notice the tightening of the muscles; feel the strain and then the release; relax and enjoy the sudden feeling of limpness.

4 ◆ You will be tensing and relaxing each muscle group twice. If any specific part of your body still feels tense after completing the exercises, go back and tense and relax those muscles again.

5 ◆ Try to keep all other muscles relaxed as you work on specific muscle groups.

6 ◆ To begin, take three deep breaths, holding each one for five to seven seconds.

7 ◆ Clench your dominant fist (right, if you are right-handed; left, if you are left-handed). Hold and count for five to seven seconds; relax. Repeat.

8 ◆ Flex your dominant bicep. Tense; relax; tense; relax.

9 ◆ Clench the fist of your nondominant hand; relax. Repeat. Proceed to the nondominant bicep. Take a couple of deep breaths and notice how relaxed and warm your arms feel. Enjoy the feeling.

10 ◆ Tense up the muscles of your forehead by raising your eyebrows as far as you can. Hold for five seconds; relax; repeat. Let the wave of relaxation cover your face.

11 ◆ Close your eyes very tightly. Release and notice the relaxation. Repeat.

12 ◆ Clench your jaws very tightly and make an exaggerated smile. Release and repeat.

13 ◆ Take a couple of deep breaths and notice how relaxed the muscles of your arms and head feel.

14 ◆ Take a deep breath and hold it for a few seconds. Release slowly. Repeat.

15 ◆ Try to touch your chin to your chest but use counterpressure to keep it from touching. Release and repeat.

16 ◆ Try to touch your back with your head, but push the opposite way with opposing muscles. Notice the tension building up. Release quickly. Repeat and let your neck become completely relaxed.

17 ◆ Push your shoulder blades back and try to make them touch. Notice the tension across your shoulders and chest. Relax and repeat.

18 ◆ Try to touch your shoulders by pushing them forward as far as you can. Hold, relax, and repeat.

19 ◆ Shrug your shoulders, trying to touch them to your ears. Hold, release, and repeat.

20 ◆ Take a very deep breath. Hold for several seconds and release slowly. Do this again, noticing the wave of relaxation overtaking your body.

21 ◆ Tighten up your stomach muscles and hold for several seconds. Release. Notice the relaxation in your abdomen. Repeat.

22 ◆ Tighten up your buttocks. Hold, release, and repeat.

23 ◆ Tense your thighs; release quickly. Repeat.

24 ◆ Point your toes away from your body; notice the tension. Return to a normal position. Repeat.

25 ◆ Point your toes toward your head; return to normal position. Repeat.

26 ◆ Point your feet outward; release quickly. Repeat.

27 ◆ Point your feet inward; hold. Relax and repeat.

28 ◆ Just let your body relax for a few minutes. Notice and enjoy the good feeling.

Practice this routine twice a day. Set a specific time for these exercises. When you feel proficient, schedule a practice for bedtime. Don't worry if you fall asleep before you finish; that's the whole point.

Other muscle relaxation approaches

There are many variations on Jacobson's relaxation technique. After some experimentation, you may develop your own. Other relaxation therapies take somewhat different approaches:

AUTOGENIC TRAINING involves concentration on standard phrases that emphasize a feeling of heaviness and relaxation in different parts of the body. For example, you imagine each extremity, one by one, as very heavy and impossible to lift.

SYSTEMATIC DESENSITIZATION involves relaxation exercises that are done before bedtime while visualizing very pleasurable, relaxing scenes. The goal is to associate bedtime with a sense of relaxation and to overcome anxiety that might interfere with sleep.

TRANSCENDENTAL MEDITATION (TM) revolves around the mental use of a sound, called a "mantra" that helps bring about a state of alert rest. The meditator sits upright with eyes closed, silently repeating the mantra as thought processes are quieted, and a state of nonthinking envelops the mind and body. During this state, oxygen consumption drops dramatically; the heartbeat slows; respiration is reduced. This technique is *not* used before sleep but during twenty-minute periods in the morning, afternoon, and evening as a prelude to activity. Its proven effectiveness in overcoming sleeplessness seems to be a carry-over from its ability to relieve daytime stress. Courses in TM are available around the country.

TM is one of the few relaxation techniques with documented efficacy. A psychologist has reported that TM helped reduce sleep latencies from more than seventy-five minutes to fifteen minutes. It also seems to increase REM periods and help sleep-deprived people return quickly to normal sleep patterns.

YOGA This ancient discipline is designed to promote physical fitness and mental well-being. Yoga is an excellent way to relax and improve your health; classes are available around the country, and there are many excellent books. To start, you might want to try these three presleep exercises:

Tension Reliever:

1 ◆ Lie flat on your back. Inhale to a count of five. Raise your arms over your head until your hands touch the bed. Make two fists.

2 ◆ Raise your buttocks. Tense and stretch every muscle in your body, including those of your face.

3 ◆ Hold for a count of five.

4 ◆ Release your breath and relax your body, keeping your arms over your head. Relax your fingers. With eyes closed, let the tension drain out of your body.

5 ◆ Slowly increase the amount of time you hold this position.

Sponge

1 ◆ Lie on your back, feet slightly apart, hands at your sides, palms upward. Close your eyes. Breathe normally.

2 ◆ Check your body for hidden tension in your legs, hands, face, shoulders.

3 ◆ Concentrate on removing all negative feelings, such as tiredness, restlessness, or tension. Mentally replace these feelings with feelings of lightness and serenity.

4 ◆ Relax each part of the body, starting at your toes and working up to your forehead. Do not rush.

Deep Breathing

1 ◆ Exhale, breathing through your nose with your mouth closed.

2 ◆ Inhale. Expand your abdomen, middle rib cage, and then the upper lungs. Hold. (Relax your face.)

3 ◆ Exhale. Release air slowly. Exhale air from the upper lungs, then from the middle rib cage. Contract your abdominal muscles slightly. Squeeze all the air out of your body.

4 ◆ Repeat six times.

Relaxing in the middle of the night (cognitive focusing)

This is a technique for getting back to sleep after awakening in the night. This simple step-by-step method was developed by two Stanford University professors of education and psychology, Thomas Coates and Carl Thoresen.

1 ◆ As soon as you realize you're awake, tell yourself something calm and reassuring, such as, "I'll fall asleep soon if I just allow myself to relax," or "I guess it's 2:00 A.M., but there's no need to worry since I'll be asleep in a few minutes."

2 ◆ Take two deep breaths and concentrate on relaxing your body. Breathe slowly in and out, imagining the tension draining out of your body. Focus on the various muscle groups (head, arms, torso, legs, and so on) so your entire body relaxes completely.

3 ◆ Take five deep breaths, counting to yourself as you take each breath. As you count, tell yourself: "I'm getting more and more calm and relaxed, peaceful and serene as I count."

4 ◆ Continue breathing deeply and focus on a pleasant mental image. Let yourself be captivated by the image. It can be a very simple one, like a flower, or it can be a beach or sunset.

5 ◆ Don't let extraneous thoughts distract you. Think of a candle flame, which flickers in the breeze that is caused by distracting thoughts. Watch the flame in your mind. Watch it become upright again as the extraneous thoughts go away, and your mind becomes ever more focused, calm, and relaxed.

Cognitive focusing is not an easy skill to master. Practice at the end of your regular bedtime relaxation sessions for several days. Don't try using it during the night until you feel that you have mastered the process. At first the results may not be dramatic. Be patient. Cognitive focusing probably will not work every time you try it, but it should help most of the time. At the very least, it can keep you from panicking when you find yourself awake in the late hours of the night.

Self-management skills

Self-management combines several specific techniques into a systematic, individualized program. It provides a complex solution to a complex problem and deals with daytime as well as nighttime concerns.

The self-management program begins with an assessment period of two to four weeks. This may include physical and neurological examination; all-night sleep recordings; psychiatric evaluation; a personal, medical, sleep, and medication history; description of sleep environment; discussion of chronic stress and tension; consideration of work demands and environments; an interview with family, spouse, and/or roommate; and a review of daily habits, including diet, caffeine use, exercise, and daily schedule.

Using this information, the therapists launch three concurrent treatment plans:

◆ *Relaxation Training*, including progressive muscle relaxation, self-hypnosis, and cognitive focusing.
◆ *"Cognitive" Restructuring*, or learning about sleep and analyzing your beliefs about sleep and your ability to sleep better.
◆ *Problem-Solving*, an analysis of the behavioral, environmental, and personal conditions related to poor sleep and design of an individualized strategy for improving sleep.

Various coping skills are evaluated and modified over the next three months. As clients work with therapists, more and more responsibility is placed on the clients to analyze continuing problems and propose and implement solutions. As part of the follow-up, therapists may bring sleep-monitoring equipment to the client's home to make all-night sleep recordings. Data on sleep, sent via telephone lines to a central computer for evaluation, provide quantitative information to check on progress.

This approach leads to changes in daytime behavior as well as nighttime sleep. As clients try to find ways to sleep better, they learn that solving any personal problem requires that they learn to view events from different perspectives. They think about past experiences in different ways and try to replace attitudes and behaviors that did not work with more suitable approaches. Clients keep careful diaries, both of nighttime sleep and of daytime stimuli that raise or lower their anxiety. They modify their work and home schedules to reduce demands on them in the evening. The underlying principle is the development of a sense of mastery and overcoming feelings of impotence in dealing with sleep problems.

This particular technique was developed at Stanford University's Stress Reduction Clinic, but similar programs are offered at other behavioral medicine centers around the country. If you are not able to participate in such projects as a patient, you can at least use some of the techniques and theories to boost your confidence in your ability to get a good night's sleep.

At Stanford, self-management skills have helped people who have suffered from sleep problems for decades, including some who were dependent on sleep medications. One teacher, who had taken nighttime medications for years, traced her sleep problems to job stress. As she learned to relax and cope better during the day, she also began to sleep better. Other participants have continued to sleep well for periods of up to five years after starting the program.

Stimulus control

This technique, developed by Richard Bootzin, a psychologist at Northwestern University, is a classic behavioral approach to sleep. It has proved to be effective by research evaluations, but it is demanding. You might want to seek the support of a sleep therapist before you use this technique.

The basic premise of stimulus control is to condition yourself to sleep when in bed. You are not allowed in bed for any purpose other than sex and sleep. Here are the fundamental guidelines:

1 ◆ Go to bed only when sleepy.
2 ◆ Do not read, eat, watch television, knit, or chat with your bed partner in bed.
3 ◆ If you don't fall asleep within ten minutes, get up and leave the bedroom.
4 ◆ Stay in the other room until you feel sleepy; then you can go back to bed.
5 ◆ If you do not fall asleep in ten minutes, get up again.
6 ◆ Do this as often as necessary until you fall asleep within ten minutes of returning to bed.
7 ◆ Regardless of how many times you commute to and from your bedroom and how little you sleep, get up at a set time.
8 ◆ Do not nap during the day.
9 ◆ Fill out a sleep log each morning. Include the number of times you went to bed and got out of bed and the total time you spent out of bed.
10 ◆ Keep careful night-by-night records.

What happens is predictable: on the first night, you may get out of bed five to ten times and get very little sleep. This might continue for several nights. This is the most difficult part of the program, since you may be tempted to give up. Turn to your therapist, family, and friends for support. If you keep conscientious records of your times in and out of bed, you should begin to see signs of progress. Within three weeks, you should be sleeping much better. In six weeks you should be able to settle down and sleep through the night.

This technique has helped people who were insomniacs for decades. Most have an occasional relapse, but complying with the sleep-in-bed-or-get-up rule helps them return to sound sleep patterns.

Stimulus control works best for people with conditioned insomnia (page 174). Often there are additional causes for their sleep problem, but resolving just one builds up confidence and often overcomes the other disturbances.

Biofeedback

Biofeedback is a method of expanding control of certain physiological functions by learning to recognize how the mind influences the body. It involves equipment that measures muscular tension or brain waves and translates these processes into audible or visual signals. By concentration, trial-and-error, and practice, a person learns how to bring about physiological changes that affect the "feedback" signal from the body.

Some psychologists explain the theory behind biofeedback by using the example of newborn babies. At birth, children cannot control the movements of their hands and flap them meaninglessly. Very quickly, infants, by watching what happens to their hands, learn how to manipulate them to carry out their wishes. But babies do not learn how to control the movements of their ears—not because it is physically impossible but because they have no way of seeing or feeling their ears move on their command.

Trained professionals use biofeedback for a wide variety of problems, including high blood pressure, tension, and sleeplessness. There are important differences in the types of biofeedback provided:

• *EMG (electromyogram) biofeedback* tunes in to the electrical currents generated by the muscles, amplifying and converting them to an audible tone. Electrodes are attached to the muscles of the forehead. Tensing the muscles raises the pitch of the tone; relaxing lowers it. Subjects hooked up to the biofeedback machine practice ways of lowering the pitch.

• *SMR (sensorimotor) biofeedback* is a method used to help a person maintain a particular electrical brain rhythm (sensorimotor rhythm) characterized by very low brain activity. This is much more difficult than learning muscle relaxation.

• *Production of theta waves*, the typical harbingers of sleep, is the goal of a third biofeedback approach that may be combined with EMG training. In most cases, researchers have found that it is far easier to learn how to suppress theta waves than it is to increase them.

Does biofeedback work for sleep problems? The answers are yes, no, and maybe.

Yes, sleep specialists have reported that people who learn to use biofeedback methods complain less about sleep difficulties and report that they fall asleep faster and sleep longer at home.

No, sleep recordings in laboratories do not always show objective improvements in sleep—even when the subjects feel that their sleep has improved. **Maybe** biofeedback works only for certain types of poor sleepers, and maybe it works in ways that cannot be measured by standard laboratory equipment.

There are definitely different success rates for EMG, SMR and theta-wave biofeedback, and it is important that the appropriate method be used for each sleep problem. Peter Hauri, Ph.D., director of Dartmouth University's sleep center and one of the nation's leading experts on biofeedback for sleep problems, has found that both EMG and SMR biofeedback can help certain patients. EMG biofeedback relieves *complaints* about sleep in people who are "hyperaroused" and have muscle tension. Easily understood, learned, and administered, EMG biofeedback is popular with patients, but laboratory findings are "less impressive" than the improvements noted on home sleep logs.

SMR biofeedback, most often used for patients who wake up often during the night, has been proved effective at home and in the laboratory. "Learning to produce more waking SMR does directly improve sleep," says Hauri. As sleep recordings verify, SMR biofeedback improves sleep efficiency (the percentage of total time in bed that is spent asleep) and lengthens NREM Stage 2 sleep. But SMR training is more difficult because the person never becomes aware of a specific SMR "feeling" or state.

Since biofeedback involves technology as well as training, technical advances may lead to greater success. A relatively inexpensive, hand-held biofeedback unit that uses skin response to help induce relaxation is available. This device might be particularly helpful for the person with sleep problems because it can be used at home where and when it is needed most. There is an additional benefit too: the unit turns itself off as soon as the user loosens his or her grip and falls asleep.

Biofeedback, while promising, is still considered an experimental approach to sleep problems. Much of the research that has been reported has involved subjects with long-standing and severe sleep disorders; success might be much greater for people with less troubled sleep patterns. Motivation is also crucial to success, because biofeedback requires a lot of practice. In most cases, a minimum of twenty minutes a day of practice was needed to help a poor sleeper fall asleep thirty minutes faster than usual. Is the daily net gain of ten minutes worth it? This is a question that you must answer for yourself.

Hypnosis

Hypnosis produces a profound change in consciousness that has often been compared to sleep, particularly to sleepwalking. Developed in the eighteenth century by Franz Mesmer, hypnosis has evolved into a widespread technique that is used for diverse purposes, from helping people overcome phobias to retrieving buried memories of crime victims.

Not everyone can be hypnotized. You must have faith in the hypnotist and be willing to heed his or her commands. Some experts have reported on successful use of hypnotic suggestions in influencing dreams, helping a person to fall asleep quickly, and preventing sleepwalking episodes. However, there is no scientific evidence from large, controlled studies to support these claims.

Some hypnotists use direct suggestion to overcome fear of insomnia and to implant a feeling of confidence and mastery in the sleeper. Some troubled sleepers play a tape recording of the hypnotist's commands at bedtime.

Some people who have problems falling asleep rely on self-hypnosis without realizing it. As they lie in bed, they tell themselves, "I am falling asleep; I am falling asleep; I am falling asleep." The fundamental principle is to think positively and believe in yourself. Sometimes such self-suggestions are combined with relaxation techniques.

Chronotherapy

More than a century ago a Scottish writer described the problem of one group of sleepless people:

"They lie awake, for perhaps two or three hours after going to bed, and do not fall into slumber until towards morning. Persons of this description often lie long and are reputed lazy by early risers, although, it is probable, they actually sleep less than these early risers themselves."

The problem—then and now—is sleep onset insomnia, caused by a biological clock that's out of synch with the rest of the world. Even a few years ago there was little that could be done to help these weary souls. However, researchers have since developed a new drug-free rescheduling treatment: chronotherapy (from the Greek word for "time").

Chronotherapy is a highly specific treatment; it will *not* work if your sleep problem is caused by anxiety or leg jerks or apnea. In selecting the first patients to undergo this treatment, sleep specialists chose only those who had experienced sleep-onset insomnia for at least three years; the insomnia also had to have a significant disrupting effect on the patient's life. An all-night sleep recording verified both the difficulty in falling asleep and otherwise normal sleep through the night. Prior to starting chronotherapy, the patients had to stop all drug use and try to maintain a very regular sleep-wake schedule, which they documented in sleep diaries. Most of the initial patients slept in a sleep laboratory during the course of treatment; however, a few successfully completed the program while sleeping at home.

The first step in chronotherapy is to impose a twenty-seven-hour "day" on the patient. If you normally fall asleep at 6:00 A.M. (even when you go to bed at midnight), you would stay up all night and go to bed at 9:00 A.M. You would sleep a normal period of time, rising at 5:00 P.M. The next day (or in some cases, a few days later) you would shift your bedtime to noon and sleep until 8:00 P.M. In the next "phase change" you would go to bed at 3:00 P.M. and wake up at 11:00 P.M.; the next phase you would sleep from 9:00 P.M. to 5:00 A.M. With the final adjustment, you would be going to bed at midnight and rising at 8:00 A.M.

This rescheduling has worked in patients who were plagued by insomnia for years and had tried dozens of other approaches. However, the key to success is to maintain the new schedule. This means no naps, no later-than-usual nights, and no sleeping in on a gloomy morning.

Chronotherapy may not work as a self-care approach to a sleep problem. Living in a world that is keeping conventional hours while you are going to bed at noon and getting up at dinner time is enormously difficult. Sleep therapists can give you the counsel and support needed to complete the rescheduling program. If you begin the treatment but do not finish or do not carry it out correctly, you may be left in a worse condition than you were before and may end up sleeping at even more undesirable hours. You also have to be motivated—from the first night that you struggle against sleepiness to stay up late to the weeks after therapy when you must adhere to a rigid sleep-wake schedule.

Psychological approaches: attributional therapy

Attributional therapy is a psychological approach for changing a poor sleeper's perception of what is causing their difficulty. Some researchers believe that sleep may improve if poor sleepers learn to attribute to themselves, rather than a pill, the ability to go to sleep easily. To test this theory, they gave insomniacs a combination treatment that included a high dose of a sleeping pill, relaxation training, and practical suggestions for improving their sleep habits. Those who slept better were divided into two groups. One group was told that the pill they had taken had been very strong and effective; the implication was that the medication had caused the improvement. The other group was told that the pill had been weak and ineffective, and that the relaxation and other therapies had helped them sleep better. The sleeping pill was then discontinued. The researchers found that the people who believed that the pill had helped them slept worse without it, while those who believed that they had helped themselves slept better.

Other psychologists have found a paradoxical effect in what they tell patients about sleep aids. When people with sleep problems were told that they were being given a stimulant at bedtime, they went to sleep quickly. When they were told they were being given a sedative, they stayed awake longer, presumably because of their anxiety about having sleep problems even after taking a sedative.

Attributional therapy has been used by trained professionals to help their clients sleep better. The purpose is not to "trick" you into sleeping better but to find ways to bolster your confidence in your ability to help yourself sleep better.

Paradoxical intention

The point of this approach is for the patient to concentrate on staying awake rather than attempting to fall asleep. This may sound like a contradictory goal, but preliminary studies show promise.

Five persons with chronic sleeplessness first tried relaxation therapies to reduce their sleep latencies, but with limited success. Then researchers at Temple University told them that their continuing problems were the result of lack of information about their presleep situation. They were told to concentrate on their thoughts before sleep and to try to remain awake as long as possible in order to describe these thoughts better. They were specifically warned that falling asleep too quickly would mean that the essential information would not be obtained.

With those instructions, the five went to bed. A woman whose initial sleep latency was 90 minutes and who had learned how to fall asleep in 70 minutes with relaxation techniques fell asleep in 5½ minutes. A man whose initial sleep latency was 57 minutes, which was reduced to 40 minutes with relaxation techniques, fell asleep in 6 minutes.

The researchers' explanation for such success is that some people react strongly to any difficulty in falling asleep. They do not see a sleep problem as an isolated event triggered by a specific factor, such as too much caffeine or stress. To them, it is a sign of a deteriorating ability to sleep, a condition that can only worsen. Because they see each night as a test of their ability to fall asleep, they become anxious at bedtime. When they do not fall asleep quickly, they start worrying about the problems that will be the result of their sleepless night. Paradoxical intention overcomes the anxiety by changing the bedtime situation. There is no need to think about performing well enough to fall asleep and so there's no anxiety. And it is much easier to sleep.

Sleep problems—like most health difficulties—are complex. Rarely is there an easy and quick solution. However, there is hope and help for troubled sleepers. The techniques in this chapter can help you start to sleep better. If you suffer from a severe sleep disorder, you may want to seek the further support and advice of a sleep specialist. Section III of this book—"Making It Through the Night"—provides basic information on what can be done about specific sleep problems, either on your own or with professional aid.

CHAPTER 10

The Perils of Sleeping Pills

C hances are you've taken sleeping pills. After aspirin, they're the most widely used drugs in the United States; some 30 million tablets are swallowed each night. This adds up to a pile of pills—600 tons—and a pile of money—110 to 175 million dollars—each year. Americans take enough sleeping pills annually to put every man, woman, and child in the nation to sleep for 200 hours.

The use of sleeping pills has become the nation's biggest drug habit. More than 20 million men and women use sleeping pills each year. And according to federal estimates, 8.5 million people—more than 5 percent of the total population—use prescription sleeping pills. Even though doctors are writing fewer prescriptions for sleep inducers than they did five or ten years ago, the total is still staggering: 25 million prescriptions a year, each for an average of forty pills. If you add the prescriptions for Valium and other common tranquilizers, which are often used to improve sleep, the total number of prescriptions for sedatives and tranquilizers is 33 million. Two-thirds are for people over the age of forty-five.

An even greater number of people buy nonprescription or over-the-counter (OTC) sleep inducers; most of these consumers are younger than forty-five. Others rely on aspirin, antihistamines, and other medications to get to sleep; the most popular sleep aid of all is alcohol.

Do all of these pill-takers and drinkers sleep better than others? Ironically, the answer is no. People who use sleeping pills regularly end up sleeping less and complaining more about sleeplessness.

Why do people take sleeping pills?

The obvious answer to this question is "to sleep better." But the real answer isn't that simple. Only 15 to 17 percent of prescriptions for sleeping pills are written for people with primary sleep disorders. According to a federal report, physicians give about 30 percent of the total sleeping pill prescriptions to people whose primary problem is psychological, almost 25 percent to patients with various medical ailments, and 18 percent to people with ill-defined, vague symptoms. If you are hospitalized, you are likely to get a sleeping pill whether or not you ask for one. At least 50 percent of all patients admitted to general hospitals each year are given sedatives or sleeping pills as a matter of routine policy. More than 20 percent of the people who become dependent on these medications acquire their drug habit in the hospital.

Many people use drugs at bedtime because they think of insomnia as a disease and a sleeping pill as a cure. Sleeplessness is a symptom, *not* an illness. Tracking down the cause of the symptom is the first step to finding any "cure." Remember that drugged sleep is not like normal sleep. You are not coping with your sleep problem by trying to overwhelm it with drugs; you are merely postponing proper treatment.

Some people expect too much from sleep. One woman thought she would look younger if she could sleep more; a man was told that his five hours of sleep a night was abnormal, and so he took pills in order to sleep longer. Others want to retreat into sleep to avoid the problems of their days. In the dark of the night, alone and weary of facing yet another difficulty, you may reach out for whatever seems easiest and simplest. It may not matter whether you intellectually recognize that the pills will not work; the need may seem too strong. The following poem, written by a accomplished poet in her seventies reveals the deep psychological needs that may make a person turn to sleeping pills:

"The light within me clicks,
Who put out the light?

"It is dark.
I am alone, afraid.
Mother, mother,
I can't sleep.

"My mother does not come.
My mother is dead.

"One pill,
Two pills,
Three pills,
Mother me, pills."

Suddenly It's Evening, Ryah Goodman, Bauhan Press, Dublin, N.H., by permission.

Recognizing why you want a pill is essential for learning to live without it—and for beginning to sleep better. Sleeping pills may seem like a simple solution, but the problems they cause are not simple.

The promise of pills

The "ideal" sleeping pill would help the user fall quickly into a normal night of restorative sleep, have no lingering aftereffects the next morning, and not be physically or psychologically addictive. This wonder drug doesn't exist; current pills do not even come close to the ideal.

None of the currently available sleeping pills induces "normal" sleep; many suppress the deepest stages of NREM sleep as well as REM sleep. Pills distort sleep stages even when taken as directed. When they are misused or overused, they destroy normal sleep. Sleep experts believe that half of patients with insomnia become worse because of sleep medication. Even after withdrawal, sleep stages may remain distorted for weeks. Ultimately, withdrawal from sleeping pills cures at least 20 percent of insomniacs.

Sleeping pills can work—but only for a very limited time. They shorten sleep latency by five to twenty minutes, decrease the number of nighttime awakenings, and extend total sleep time. The effects of most pills wear off in three to seven nights. Then—as confirmed both by subjective report and objective sleep recordings—the pill user takes just as long to fall asleep, wakes up as often, and sleeps no longer than someone with the same problem who has not taken any pills. The longest-working sleepin is Dalmane (flurazepam), a prescription drug that has been proved in limited studies to extend total sleep time for up to twenty-eight days.

The problems with pills

As a lasting solution to a sleep problem, sleeping pills do little, if any, good. And they can do considerable harm.

A major study of health habits demonstrated that people who used sleeping pills regularly faced a 50 percent higher risk of death. Sleep drugs are the third most common means of suicide, and they are implicated in a third of all drug-related deaths, intentional and accidental, each year. The newer pills, like Dalmane, generally are not used as a means of suicide. However, they can be especially hazardous when combined with alcohol. There also is a risk of accidental overdose by other family members, such as children.

The chart on page 134 summarizes the most common dangers of sleeping pill use. Certain people are so vulnerable to potential risks that they should *never* use any sleeping pill. They are:

• People with chronic breathing problems, particularly sleep apnea (pages 192 and 227), because sleeping pills further depress the body's ability to breathe. If you suspect you have a nocturnal breathing problem, if you have chronic lung disease, or if you know that you're a loud, vigorous snorer, stay away from pills.

• People with impaired kidneys or livers. Since many sleeping pills pass through these organs, a dysfunction may mean that the drugs stay in the body for a much longer time than is usual.

• People taking medications for medical illness or chronic disease. The use of sleeping pills can lead to harmful, even life-threatening interactions with other drugs and can affect the way other drugs are metabolized.

• Pregnant women, because sleeping pills, like other drugs, may affect their unborn children. The most notorious example of this problem was the use of Thalidomide, a sedative that caused severe birth defects. Other sleeping pills have been associated with cardiovascular abnormalities and problems such as cleft palates in newborns.

• Older adults, who are at risk for several reasons. They are more likely to have serious medical problems, to be taking other medications, and to have impaired respiration at night; their bodies may require more time to break down and eliminate drugs. Also, when older persons wake up confused, agitated, and delusional from drugged sleep, there is a risk that they may physically harm themselves.

• Anyone who has been drinking. The effects of sleeping pills and alcohol are increased, sometimes with deadly results, when ingested together. A comparatively small amount of a sleeping pill can lead to a fatal overdose in an alcoholic.

You should also be mindful of *when* you take a sleeping pill. If you take a pill right after a heavy meal, you will not feel any effect immediately. If you take another pill, both may hit you at the same time, producing excessive and prolonged depression of your central nervous system. Antacids also affect the absorption of sleeping pills in your body. So, it is important that you take a sleeping pill only when your stomach is empty.

Evaluating sleeping pills

Even the earliest civilizations brewed up sleep potions, herbal teas, and soporific ointments for the sake of a good night's sleep. Folk remedies, ranging from malted milk to bone meal tablets to cider vinegar and honey, still abound. But you expect something more from marketed sleep remedies: proof that they will live up to their promises. However, the history of modern sleep aids is a story of unfulfilled expectations.

The barbiturates, developed at the turn of the century, promised to be modern medicine's first major advance in sleep medications. However, the dangers of tolerance, dependence, and overdose in these drugs eventually overshadowed their therapeutic benefits. Since then each new sleep drug has been heralded with great enthusiasm as a safer, more effective alternative. After the burst of initial excitement, each bright new hope has faded. The benzodiazepines, produced in the fifties, represented a new generation of sleeping pills and tranquilizers. One of these drugs, Dalmane, has become the most popular sleep medication in the country. However, recent evidence indicates that Dalmane has lingering and significant effects on daytime performance. Shorter-acting benzodiazepines that stay in the body for a few hours rather than a few days are currently being tested.

One problem in evaluating all sleeping pills is in measuring improvement of a disorder that is often only vaguely defined. Laboratory research is done on healthy, young volunteers who may have no sleep complaints or on people with severe, chronic problems. There are no long-term studies to determine the effects of years of intermittent or regular use and no complete assessments of daytime functioning and mood as well as nighttime sleep.

Scientists know even less about over-the-counter products than they do about prescription sleeping pills. In the mid-1970s the primary ingredient in nonprescription sleep inducers, an antihistamine called methapyrilene, was banned by the Food and Drug Administration (FDA) as a suspected carcinogen. In issuing tentative guidelines on currently available OTC sleep aids, the FDA has found *none* that it deemed safe and effective.

The Dangers of Sleeping Pills

1 ◆ Fatal overdoses, particularly if combined with alcohol and other drugs that act on the central nervous system
2 ◆ Harmful interactions with other drugs prescribed for medical problems
3 ◆ Dangerous, even life-threatening interference with respiration in people with chronic breathing problems
4 ◆ "Hangover" effects that impair daytime coordination, driving skills, logical thinking, and mood
5 ◆ Development of physical and/or psychological dependence
6 ◆ Development of tolerance so that the initial dose stops working
7 ◆ Exacerbation of the initial sleep problem
8 ◆ Disruption of normal sleep stages
9 ◆ Harmful effects on people who have chronic medical problems, particularly ailments of the kidneys, liver, or lungs
10 ◆ Confusion, hallucinations, and other adverse effects in the elderly
11 ◆ If taken in pregnancy, possible birth defects for the child
12 ◆ Difficulty awakening to respond to a fire alarm, crying child, or other crisis

Adapted from *Sleeping Pills, Insomnia and Medical Practice*, 1979, with the permission of the National Academy of Sciences, Washington, D.C.

Sleep Sense

Understanding sleeping pills

The following information on specific drugs is important because not all sleeping pills are alike or act alike in the body. Here is some essential information on the way in which drugs function in the body:

• *Half-life.* This term refers to the amount of time it takes for *half* of the amount of drug you ingested to leave your body. If a drug has a short half-life of three hours, this means that half of the amount you took is still in your body three hours later. Drugs with long half-lives are more troubling: half of the active ingredients in a sleeping pill with a half-life of fifty hours remains in your body for more than two days after you swallow it. Sleeping pills with long half-lives are likely to impair your daytime functioning and mood.

• *Drug Interactions.* Different medications or chemicals may combine within your body to enhance, slow, or oppose each other's effects. Alcohol and sleeping pills, taken together, have a much greater impact on the central nervous system than either substance taken alone. Sleeping pills also may interact with other drugs taken for medical problems and may produce unexpected and dangerous complications.

• *Method of Elimination.* If you know how a drug is eliminated from your body and how much of it leaves unchanged, you can identify the organs involved in processing the substance. The liver and kidneys play vital roles in clearing many sleeping pills from the body, and any malfunction of these organs may slow the normal time in which these drugs are eliminated. A drug that is excreted virtually unchanged will have less of an impact within the body than one that is fully metabolized.

A guide to sleeping prescription pills

Barbiturates (Seconal, Amytal, Nembutal, Tuinal)

Some 2,500 types of barbiturates have been developed since 1903; about 50 have been marketed for medical use. The 12 in current use are prescribed as hypnotics, antianxiety agents, anesthetics, and anticonvulsants.

Barbiturates are often classified by the duration of their action in the body. Short-acting barbiturates, such as Brevital (methohexital), have half-lives of three to eight hours and are used primarily as anesthetics injected into the blood vessels. Butisol (butobarbital) and phenobarbital are used mainly as anticonvulsants and antianxiety drugs.

The barbiturates most commonly used as sleeping pills are: Seconal (secobarbital), which has a half-life of twenty to twenty-eight hours; Amytal (amobarbital), with a half-life of fourteen to forty-two hours; Nembutal (pentobarbital), with a half-life of twenty-one to forty-two hours; and Tuinal, a combination of amobarbital and secobarbital. The barbiturates are processed more quickly if taken repeatedly because they stimulate liver enzymes that initiate drug metabolism.

IN THE BODY Barbiturates are salts that are rapidly absorbed from the intestinal tract. The longer-acting ones used as sleeping pills are excreted partially unchanged in the liver. Because these drugs stimulate the liver enzymes, they increase the liver's metabolic rate, not only of themselves but of a wide range of other drugs. Thus, barbiturates can diminish the effectiveness of normal doses of such medications as anticoagulants (taken by people to prevent the development of blood clots) and antidepressants.

BENEFITS/RISKS Barbiturates can temporarily induce and extend sleep with little "hangover" effect the next day. However, they are considered to be extremely hazardous because they can rapidly lead to tolerance and dependence, and they are dangerous, even deadly, when misused. Barbiturates also disrupt the normal sleep cycle by suppressing REM and deep NREM sleep.

A dose that is approximately ten times the usual sleep-inducing dosage of .1 gram can produce serious side effects; fifteen to twenty times the therapeutic dose can be lethal. Alcohol drastically increases the dangers, and much lower doses of barbiturates may be deadly if taken with alcohol. Because of the severe liver damage associated with alcoholism, an alcoholic may be unusually sensitive to barbiturates. The symptoms of barbiturate overdose include respiratory depression, kidney failure, circulatory malfunctioning, and coma. There is no specific antidote for an overdose; however, mortality in patients who are brought to emergency rooms alive is only one percent, primarily because of the effectiveness of modern resuscitation techniques.

If taken for prolonged periods, barbiturates lead to physical dependence.

Addiction typically occurs if a person has been taking doses that are four to eight times the minimum therapeutic dose for two to eight months. During withdrawal, sleep becomes more disturbed than before the drug was first used. In addition to REM rebound and frightening hallucinations, the ex-user is likely to experience tremulousness, anxiety, sleeplessness, and in severe cases, delirium and seizures.

CURRENT USAGE Prescriptions for barbiturates have dropped markedly in the last two decades because of the dangers of overdose and dependence and the development of safer drugs. In 1971, 47 percent of the prescriptions for hypnotic drugs were for barbiturates; by 1977, only 17 percent were. During the same time period, there has been a 52 percent decline in the number of barbiturate suicides.

Benzodiazepines (Dalmane, Valium, Librium)

In the past two decades, benzodiazepines have had an enormous impact on drug use. Valium (diazepam) is the most commonly prescribed medication in the Western world; millions of people rely on its tranquilizing and muscle-relaxing effects daily. Librium (chlordiazepoxide) is a widely used sedative, muscle-relaxant, and anticonvulsant drug. Altogether, 2,000 benzodiazepines have been synthesized, and a large number are used clinically. Only one is used specifically as a hypnotic in this country: Dalmane (flurazepam), the most widely prescribed sleeping medication in the United States. Valium and, to a lesser extent, Librium are often taken at bedtime as sleep-inducers.

IN THE BODY Benzodiazepines are primarily metabolized by the liver and are excreted by the kidneys. The commonly used ones, which have long half-lives, break down into powerful metabolites (by-products) that act on the brain. Dalmane produces the metabolite called N_1-desalkyl-flurazepam, which has the longest half-life of the benzodiazepine by-products: 47 to 100 hours. It also tends to build up in the body with successive nightly use. This is why Dalmane seems to work better on the second or third night rather than the first night it is used and why it continues to be effective on the first night it is *not* used. By the seventh to tenth morning after consecutive nightly doses, the accumulated levels of Dalmane are four to six times higher than on the first morning; these are daytime as well as nighttime levels. With continued use, people taking Dalmane may have as much of the drug in their bloodstream during the day, when they are trying to work, as during the night, when they are hoping to rest.

Unlike the barbiturates, the benzodiazepines do not interfere with the metabolism of other drugs. However, their elimination from the body is greatly impaired and slowed in the elderly and in people with liver diseases.

BENEFITS/RISKS Taken as directed, Dalmane decreases sleep latency, reduces body movements and awakenings in the night, and lowers the number of shifts in sleep stages. Total sleep time and Stage 2 NREM sleep are increased; deep NREM sleep and, to a lesser extent, REM are decreased. Since Valium is not prescribed as a hypnotic, it has not been evaluated for its sleep-enhancing properties. However, it seems to improve the ability to fall asleep and stay asleep during initial use.

Dalmane has been proved effective for a longer period of time than other sleeping pills—up to twenty-eight nights. However, only ten people were involved in this long-term study; other studies of Dalmane's efficacy have been for shorter periods.

There is an increased risk of birth defects if Dalmane or Valium is taken during pregnancy. They also are not recommended for use by children because of the lack of clinical testing. Given during childbirth, Valium has been linked to respiratory difficulties in the newborn.

Suicide through the use of benzodiazepines is uncommon, and the few reported deaths have been attributed to doses that were five to nineteen times above the normal therapeutic dose of fifteen to thirty milligrams of Dalmane or two to ten milligrams of Valium. However, there are increasing reports of accidental or intentional deaths caused by a combination of benzodiazepines and alcohol.

Scientists do not understand the physiological basis for the strong interaction between alcohol and the benzodiazepines, but their combined and enhanced effect on behavior and perception is undeniable. Daytime functioning is *more* impaired by a combination of alcohol and benzodiazepines than by combinations of other sleeping pills and alcohol. Taken with alcohol, Dalmane impairs performance in simulated driving tests and alters coordination, reaction time, and judgment. People who took Dalmane and alcohol ignored driving rules and made serious steering errors; they were completely unaware of their diminished ability. These problems were compounded if they also took Valium during the day. The loss of inhibition and poor judgment were also obvious in social situations.

Even the most sober of Dalmane users experience some decrement in daytime functioning, including problems in concentration, manual dexterity, and judgment. In some studies, Dalmane had the same effects as alcohol on aggression and discretion. In a test of many substances that affect behavior, Dalmane led to the most severe changes in behavior, including a murder threat, uncharacteristic weeping, quarreling, and a car crash.

Driving and operating machinery seem particularly hazardous for someone who is using Dalmane, primarily because chronic users do not realize how poorly they are functioning. In one study of the use of Dalmane over a three-week period, the subjects recognized that their skills were impaired during the first week, but by the third week, when they were doing much more poorly, they were no longer able to perceive the changes in their functioning. Other studies have shown that the effects of Dalmane do not "wear off" during the day; volunteers performed poorly on tests given in the morning, midday, and late afternoon.

Regular use of benzodiazepines for sleep can lead to psychological dependence, if not physical addiction. If a person has been taking three to five times the normal dosage for several months, withdrawal can trigger seizures and delirium. Mild withdrawal symptoms may occur even after the use of minimal therapeutic doses. In the elderly, there seems to be additional risk of confusion and agitation during nights in which benzodiazepines are used.

CURRENT USAGE More than half of all the sleeping pill prescriptions written in the United States today are for Dalmane—more than 13 million prescriptions a year. Physicians tend to choose Dalmane because it seems less dangerous than the barbiturates, with less risk of abuse, addiction, and difficult withdrawal.

However, physicians are troubled by the fact that Dalmane builds up in the body, and they are often hesitant to prescribe it for elderly persons, whose metabolism is slower acting. Many authorities are recommending that nightly dosages for all users be reduced by half—to fifteen milligrams—to diminish the problem of daytime impairments. Users are also being warned about the dangers of driving and operating machinery after taking Dalmane.

Chloral hydrate (NOCTEC)

Chloral hydrate, sold by its generic name as well as by the brand name *Noctec*, is the oldest hypnotic in use. It is perhaps most famous—or more precisely, infamous—as one of the ingredients in a "Mickey Finn," a knockout drink mixed with alcohol.

IN THE BODY Chloral hydrate is rapidly metabolized and produces trichlorethanol, a metabolite with a half-life of six to eight hours that breaks down into other byproducts which are excreted in urine or bile. One of these metabolites, trichloroacetic acid, stimulates the liver to metabolize other drugs more quickly and may increase the action of certain anticoagulant medications.

Chloral hydrate seems to act primarily on the brain with little depression of blood pressure or respiration. There is no "hangover" the next morning.

BENEFITS/RISKS Chloral hydrate produces drowsiness, followed by sleep within an hour. The therapeutic dose (500 milligrams-1 gram) produces few side-effects and has no significant effects on daytime performance.

Chloral hydrate can be habit-forming if taken regularly. However, dependence has become much less of a problem since the 1800s, when chloral hydrate was a popular drug of abuse. Because of its effect on anticoagulant medications, it is prescribed only with great caution for patients receiving such drugs. It is also not given to patients with impaired kidney or liver function.

Chloral hydrate is used for patients who cannot take other prescription sleep aids, including the young, the elderly, and the ill. It is often used as a preoperative sedative and as a postoperative sleep aid along with pain-relieving drugs.

Overdoses of four to ten times the therapeutic dosage may result in severe and sometimes lethal complications. The symptoms of overdose are similar to those with barbiturates, but there is an added risk of irregular heart rhythms and permanent damage to liver or kidneys. Alcohol drastically increases the dangers of use and overuse of chloral hydrate.

CURRENT USAGE With the advent of the benzodiazepines, chloral hydrate went out of fashion as a hypnotic. However, because overdoses and deaths are now rare, some clinicians are choosing it over Dalmane for patients who might be at risk because of Dalmane's lingering effects in the body.

Triclos (triclofos sodium)

Triclos (triclofos sodium) is related to chloral hydrate and has many of the same properties and effects.

IN THE BODY Triclos rapidly produces high levels of trichlorethanol—the same metabolite obtained from chloral hydrate—in the blood; peak levels are reached in an hour. The half-life is approximately eleven hours.

Triclos—like chloral hydrate—may affect the metabolism of other drugs, primarily anticoagulants, in the liver.

BENEFITS/RISKS Triclos induces sleep quickly, diminishes nocturnal awakenings, and extends sleep time. It has not been shown to be effective for more than fourteen days.

Triclos may be habit-forming. It is prescribed only with great caution for people taking anticoagulants or those with cardiac arrhythmias or severe heart disease.

It may reduce alertness and should not be taken before driving or operating machinery. Alcohol and tranquilizers greatly enhance its effects on the central nervous system. The therapeutic dosage is 1500 milligrams; overdose is possible, and the symptoms resemble those of barbiturate overdose.

CURRENT USAGE Triclos' use is similar to that of chloral hydrate.

Placidyl (ethchlorvynol)

Placidyl (ethchlorvynol) is a widely used prescription sleeping pill that is chemically unrelated to the barbiturates, the benzodiazepines, and other hypnotic drugs.

IN THE BODY Placidyl is rapidly absorbed from the digestive tract and is almost completely metabolized by the body. Only .1 percent is excreted unchanged in the urine. Placidyl reaches peak blood levels in two hours and has a short half-life of six hours. Few data are available on its metabolism and effects on the liver.

BENEFITS/RISKS Placidyl improves sleep onset, and its sleep-inducing effects last for about five hours. However, it remains effective for only a short period of time.

Placidyl is not recommended for pregnant women, children, people who are taking anticoagulant drugs, patients with impaired kidney or liver function, and elderly or debilitated patients.

Dependence is a major risk and can occur with continued use of only two or three times the therapeutic dose (500 milligrams). Even one gram a day has led to signs and symptoms of intoxication, including lack of coordination, tremors, confusion, slurred speech, and muscle weakness. Withdrawal may trigger convulsions, delirium, perceptual disorders, memory loss, tremors, nausea, vomiting, and twitching.

Overdoses are characterized by prolonged deep coma, decreased respiration and heart rate, and a drop in blood pressure. There is great variation in reactions to the drug; people who have taken 14 times the therapeutic dose have died, while others have survived after taking 120 times that amount.

CURRENT USAGE Although Placidyl is widely prescribed, a report of the National Academy of Sciences stated that it had "only weak and short-lived effects on sleep in laboratory studies. Recently, it was reported to cause confusion and emotional distress the next day."

Quaalude, Mequin, Sopor (methaqualone)

Quaalude, Mequin, and Sopor are brand names for the chemical methaqualone, which is used as an anticonvulsant, local anesthetic, and antihistamine as well as a hypnotic.

IN THE BODY A white, crystalline powder with a bitter taste, methaqualone is highly soluble in water and is rapidly absorbed from the digestive tract. It quickly reaches peak doses in the body but has a moderately long half-life of eighteen to forty-two hours; one recent study reported that its half-life can be as long as seventy hours. It is metabolized in the liver, and its by-products are excreted in urine and feces.

BENEFITS/RISKS Methaqualone induces sleep within thirty minutes and provides sleep that lasts for five to eight hours with little "hangover" the next morning. It has not been proven effective for more than fourteen nights.

Methaqualone is believed to cause birth defects if taken by pregnant women; it is not recommended for use by children. Tolerance develops quickly, and chronic use leads to physical and psychological dependence.

This substance is often abused; the pills are sold on the street as "quads" and are used as downers. Even a month of overuse can trigger withdrawal symptoms. Taken with alcohol or other depressants of the central nervous system, methaqualone affects performance and respiration. Acute overdosage may result in restlessness, convulsions, delirium, and coma, and may be fatal.

CURRENT USAGE Methaqualone is not a preferred sleep aid because of the dangers of abuse, dependence, and overdose.

Doriden (glutethimide)

Introduced in 1954 as a potential replacement for barbiturates, Doriden— more commonly referred to by its generic name, glutethimide—has proved to be just as toxic and addictive. It is classified as one of a group of drugs called the "piperidinediones."

IN THE BODY Glutethimide is absorbed poorly and somewhat erratically from the intestinal tract. A white, crystalline powder, it is practically insoluble in water. Peak concentrations in the blood occur from one to six hours after ingestion; the average half-life in the blood is ten to twelve hours. It is metabolized by the liver and can stimulate the liver enzymes, affecting the way other drugs are metabolized. It can block the passage of certain nerve impulses, interfering with basic functions such as digestion.

BENEFITS/RISKS Glutethimide has been proved to be an effective hypnotic for three to seven days. It may impair the ability to drive or perform other hazardous activities requiring mental alertness or physical coordination. The usual adult dosage is .25 to .5 gram at bedtime. Doses from 10 to 20 grams have proved to be lethal. A single dose of 5 grams usually produces severe intoxication. Respiration depression is less severe than with barbiturates, but the effects on the heart may be greater. Muscle spasms and convulsions may occur. Characteristically, a person who has taken an overdose may appear to recover from a coma and then lapse into unconsciousness again. In those who take deliberate overdoses, the mortality rate is thirteen times higher than for barbiturate users who reach the emergency room alive. In one series of 208 nonnarcotic drug overdoses, glutethimide led to the greatest number of deaths.

CURRENT USAGE Because of its serious dangers of addiction and overdose, glutethimide is not often used as a sleeping pill. Many doctors feel that its hazards are so grave that it should not be prescribed under any circumstances.

Noludar (Methyprylon)

Noludar, more commonly referred to by its generic name, methyprylon, belongs to the same family as Doriden (glutethimide) and presents many of the same disadvantages.

IN THE BODY A white, crystalline powder, methyprylon is soluble in water. It reaches peak levels in the bloodstream one to two hours after ingestion. Most of the drug is metabolized in the body; only three percent is passed unchanged in the urine.

BENEFITS/RISKS Methyprylon reduces sleep latency time in most insomniacs and provides sleep for five to eight hours for a period of seven nights.

Combined with alcohol, it has a more drastic impact on the central nervous system. Overdoses are very dangerous and often fatal. However, the mortality rate is not as high as with glutethimide. There also seems to be great variation in individual reactions to this drug. There have been reports of deaths in people who took fifteen times the normal therapeutic dose (300 to 400 milligrams), while others have survived amounts sixty times above this level.

CURRENT USAGE Because of its risks, methyprylon is rarely used as a sleep aid.

Other prescription drugs used as sleep inducers

Antihistamines

Histamine is a chemical substance normally released by specific cells in the skin and mucous membranes when they are irritated or injured. The release of histamine characterizes allergic reactions, such as itching, swelling, hay fever, and asthma. Antihistamines, as their name implies, are drugs that counter histamine's noxious effects. One of their most common side-effects is drowsiness, and this is why they are used—or more precisely, misused—as sleep inducers. While many people think of them as somehow safer or milder than true hypnotics, there is no scientific data to confirm this belief.

The appeal of antihistamines is their short half-life. Within an hour of administration, they reach peak concentrations in body tissues and are rapidly metabolized by the liver. They seem to be completely absent from the body in six hours, and there is no known potential for addiction. The most commonly used prescription antihistamine is Benadryl (dephenhydramine), which is used for allergies, motion sickness, Parkinson's disease, and as an adjunct in treatment of psychiatric patients with anxiety. Like other antihistamines, it is far from being risk-free. Side-effects include dizziness, lack of coordination, blurred vision, nervousness, loss of appetite, frequent urination, skin rashes, headache, nausea, vomiting, tightness of the chest, and wheezing and cardiac irregularities. Massive overdoses can be fatal.

It is always risky to use a medicine for a purpose other than for what it was intended. You should be cautious about using antihistamines, as you should be about any hypnotic; and be particularly wary of combining the two—severe complications are the result.

Antipsychotic drugs

The powerful medications for serious mental illness are sometimes used to relieve nighttime agitation, particularly in elderly psychiatric patients. Fatal overdoses are rare, but there are severe side-effects, including tardive dyskinesia—the loss of control of the facial and mouth muscles. The use of these medications for insomnia has been questioned and criticized.

Antidepressant drugs

Different types of antidepressants have different effects on sleep. The ones most commonly used for nighttime sedation are Elavil (amitriptyline), Adapin (doxepin), and Sinequan (doxepin). The basis for their sedating effects is unclear, but there is no known potential for dependence. Like all antidepressant medications, they are effective only in patients with severe depression. Overdoses, with amounts as low as six times the therapeutic dose, can be lethal. These drugs should only be taken under the close supervision of a psychiatrist.

Over-the-counter nonprescription sleep aids

It looks so easy in the television commercials: the actor takes a tablet or two of a well-known medication available at any drugstore, yawns, shuts off the light, and falls asleep.

The appeal of such seemingly easy sleep is so strong that more than 5 percent of all American adults purchase nonprescription sleep aids each year.

There is no question that over-the-counter (OTC) sleeping pills are very big business. But are they good medicine? Can you be sure that the drugs you are taking at bedtime are safe and effective?

The answer from the Food and Drug Administration (FDA) is no. After a detailed, comprehensive review of the ingredients of the major nonprescription sleep aids, the FDA issued tentative guidelines stating that *none* of the active ingredients in these products meet their criteria for safety and efficacy.

The FDA concluded that the following ingredients in OTC preparations are "not generally recognized as safe and effective or are misbranded":

• *Bromides*: ammonium bromides, potassium bromide, and sodium bromide. These drugs displace the normal chloride ion in the body with a bromide ion, causing depression of the central nervous system. They also tend to accumulate in the body when used regularly and thus pose a serious hazard to health.

• *Methapyrilene hydrochloride and methapyrilene fumarate*: There is considerable evidence that these medications may be effective in inducing sleep, but they present a potential danger so significant that it overrides the question of efficacy: they are carcinogenic. Methapyrilene has been identified as a factor in the development of cancer in laboratory rats. The data is not conclusive, however. Another possible side-effect of these drugs is interference with the brain impulses that regulate basic body functions.

• *Scopolamine. compounds*—scopolomine aminoxide hydrobromide and scopolamine hydrobromide: Scopolamine occurs naturally as a derivative of belladonna, or deadly nightshade. The scopolamine compounds are street drugs that are widely abused. Even in relatively small doses, they can cause serious complications, such as dangerous states of delusion similar to psychosis. Other side-effects include: dryness of the mouth, blurred vision, abnormal intolerance of light, cardiac effects, acute glaucoma, constipation, urinary retention, movement disorders, and problems of body temperature regulation.

• *Miscellaneous compounds*: acetaminophen (Tylenol), aspirin, passionflower extract, salicylamides and thiamine (Vitamin B_1) hydrochloride. There is a lack of valid scientific data on the efficacy of these agents as sleep aids.

As a result of these findings, the FDA has ordered changes in the advertising for sleeping pills containing these ingredients. No longer can the packages state that the drugs "help you relax so you can fall asleep," or are "non-habit-forming" or "guaranteed fast acting," or produce sleep that is "natural," "normal," or "sound."

◆ *Nonprescription Antihistamines*: The FDA recognizes antihistamines as a separate group because "the available data are insufficient to permit final classification at this time." Introduced originally for the relief of hay fever and allergic reactions, they produce drowsiness as a side-effect. In higher dosages, antihistamines are often used to induce sleep (see page 144). However, there is little evidence that the much lower doses of antihistamines in OTC sleep aids have any impact on sleep.

The most common antihistamine used in OTC sleep aids is pyrilamine maleate. Some scientists believe that this agent may be similar to methapyrilene, the antihistamine that was banned because it caused cancer in laboratory rats. OTC sleep aids contain a very low level—twenty-five milligrams—of this substance, and the FDA is continuing tests for both safety and efficacy. Also under investigation are other antihistamines, including diphenhydramine hydrochloride, doxylamine succinate, and phenyltoloxamine dihydrogen citrate.

Only one OTC product contains one of the antihistamines listed above: Unisom, with the active ingredient doxylamine succinate. Its manufacturer reports that Unisom compares favorably to prescription barbiturate drugs (page 135) in shortening sleep latency. In studies with placebos, doxylamine succinate shortened sleep latency by a third and extended sleep by 26 percent. However, as a consumer you should keep in mind that this drug was reviewed under the regulations for new drug applications, which guarantee confidentiality of submitted test results, and so it has not undergone the same public review as the other OTC sleep aids.

Overdoses with antihistamines can be dangerous, resulting in nausea, vomiting, feverishness, excitability, hallucinations, and convulsions. In severe cases, coma and cardiorespiratory collapse may occur. Emergency treatment is crucial.

The chart on page 150 lists the most common OTC sleep aids, their ingredients and their potential dangers.

Aspirin

Aspirin, the "wonder drug," is the most widely used medication in the world. If taken occasionally at bedtime, it can help you fall asleep. This was the finding of researchers at the sleep center at Dartmouth Medical School. In studies of people who have severe insomnia, two tablets of aspirin helped them fall asleep quickly and sleep through the night with fewer awakenings. Sleep recordings showed that aspirin has no effect on sleep stages or REM periods, but it seems to have more impact in maintaining sleep during the second half of the night.

Aspirin, like other sleep-inducing drugs, provides only temporary benefits. Its ability to induce sleep wears in three nights. And like other sleep drugs, withdrawal from the drug after chronic use can lead to sleeplessness.

L-tryptophan

L-tryptophan is an amino acid—a natural agent, not a drug—found within the body and in many foods, including milk products and tuna. Since it is not a medication, it is not governed or evaluated by the Food and Drug Administration, and it is available without prescription at most large health food stores.

L-tryptophan has been heralded in many lay publications as nature's own sleeping pill, the ultimate cure for insomnia. Scientists have been more cautious in their evaluations, but they also believe that tryptophan may be an effective and safe sleep aid.

Dr. Ernest Hartmann and his colleagues at Tufts University, who have done most of the available research on L-tryptophan, concluded that it can reduce sleep latency from twenty minutes to ten minutes, in doses of one to ten grams.

L-tryptophan should be taken at least forty-five minutes before you want to fall asleep because it works more slowly than some other sleep inducers. Low doses are well tolerated, and there are few reports of complications. However, some people have experienced nausea and vomiting after ingesting high doses.

Research on the safety and efficacy of this substance is continuing, and scientists are wary of potential dangers: one concern is that bladder cancer has been detected in rats given L-tryptophan, but this finding is disputed. Another concern is that extra amounts of an amino acid might affect protein synthesis.

Tryptophan is rapidly synthesized and eliminated from the body; it has little effect on sleep stages. Scientists believe that it induces sleep because it is one of the building blocks of serotonin, the brain chemical associated with sleep.

Tryptophan, like other substances, is not a panacea and is not recommended for regular use. It should not be viewed as a "cure" for sleeplessness but, rather, as one means of coping as you work toward a lasting solution to your sleep problems.

Some people have suggested that drinking milk or eating foods rich in tryptophan before bedtime can help you to fall asleep faster. While milk is a soothing nightcap, you should realize that it contains far too little tryptophan to affect your sleep. You would have to drink more than half a dozen glasses of milk before the amount of tryptophan would be sufficient to induce sleep.

Breaking the habit

Withdrawal from sleeping pills can be as difficult as withdrawal from narcotics. Often a chronic user is both physiologically and psychologically addicted. Many people take several drugs in different amounts and at different times. Sudden withdrawal after erratic and prolonged use can lead to many serious symptoms, including severe insomnia, extreme anxiety, stomach cramps, nausea, vomiting, weakness, rapid breathing, fear, hallucinations, dehydration, convulsions, uncontrollable twitching, hypertension, and terrifying nightmares.

Quitting "cold turkey" after long reliance on sleeping pills is risky, and you should never try to do it alone. Most physicians will begin by stabilizing your sleeping pill regimen at a consistent nightly dose. You will be instructed to take the same dose at the same time each night. The withdrawal rate will be slow and steady, usually a decrease of one therapeutic dose (for example, one milligram) a week. If you have been taking several drugs, only one will be withdrawn at a time.

At each step, you should anticipate some sleep problems. If the pills have been suppressing REM periods, you should be prepared for vivid—sometimes bizarre—nightmares. The poor sleep and bad dreams are not permanent; they are temporary signs that you are weaning yourself from the powerful drugs. If you are discouraged, talk to your physician or sleep therapist. Try charting your progress to keep up your motivation.

The final step is complete drug withdrawal. Your sleep should continue to improve gradually over a four to six-week period. It is possible that your original sleep problem, long masked by drugs, will resurface. This time, seek out proper help in dealing with it. Withdrawal alone "cures" a fifth of reported cases of insomnia and improves half of all sleep complaints.

Over-the-Counter Nonprescription Sleep Aids

Brand name (manufacturer)	Active ingredients per tablet	How drug acts in the body	Dosage	Manufacturer's warnings
NERVINE (Miles)	25 milligrams (mg) pyrilamine maleate (antihistamine)	Antihistamine acts on central nervous system to produce drowsiness	2 tablets at bedtime; Maximum—4 every 24 hrs.	Not for prolonged use. Do not use in children under 12, if pregnant or nursing, if you have asthma, glaucoma, or enlarged prostate gland. Seek immediate treatment in case of overdose. Do not use if you have been using alcohol.
NYTOL	25 mg. pyrilamine maleate (antihistamine)	Antihistamine acts on central nervous system to induce drowsiness.	1 or 2 tablets 20 minutes before bedtime	Not for prolonged use. Not for use by children, women who are pregnant or nursing, men with enlarged prostate glands, people with asthma or glaucoma. Take with caution if drinking alcohol. Do not take if using other drugs except under physician's supervision.
QUIET WORLD (Whitehall)	162 mg. acetaminophen 227 mg. aspirin 25 mg. pyrilamine maleate (antihistamine)	Aspirin and acetaminophen (Tylenol) relieve pain or headache due to cold, flu, sinus pain, muscle aches, menstrual cramps; antihistamine induces drowsiness.	2 tablets at bedtime; maximum—4.	Not for prolonged use. Do not use in children under 12, if pregnant or nursing, if under medical care. Consult physician if pain persists for more than 10 days or if redness is present. Do not drive or operate machinery after use.

Product	Active Ingredient	Action	Dosage	Cautions
SLEEP-EZE (*Whitehall*)	25 mg. pyrilamine maleate (antihistamine)	Antihistamine acts on central nervous system to induce drowsiness.	1 or 2 tablets at bedtime; maximum—4.	Not for prolonged use. Do not use in children under 12, if pregnant or nursing, if you are presently taking a prescription or other nonprescription drug unless directed by physician. Take with caution if alcohol has been consumed.
SOMINEX (*Williams*)	25 mg. pyrilamine maleate (antihistamine)	Antihistamine acts on central nervous system to induce drowsiness.	2 tablets at bedtime.	Not for prolonged use. Do not use in children under 12, if suffering from glaucoma, asthma, or enlarged prostrate, if pregnant or nursing. Depression of central nervous system is enhanced by alcohol and other hypnotic drugs.
UNISOM (*Leming Division Pfizer*)	25 mg. dolylamine succinate 2-(a-(2-dimethylaminoethoxy)-a-methylbenzyl) pyridine succinate (antihistamine)	This antihistamine (of the ethanolamine class) acts on the central nervous system to induce drowsiness	1 tablet 30 minutes before retiring.	Do not take for more than 2 weeks. Not for use in children, if pregnant or nursing, if you have asthma, glaucoma, or enlarged prostate. Do not take without physician's approval if you are taking any other drug. Use with caution if alcohol has been consumed.

[NOTE: All other currently available OTC sleep aids rely on the same primary ingredient, pyrilamine maleate.]

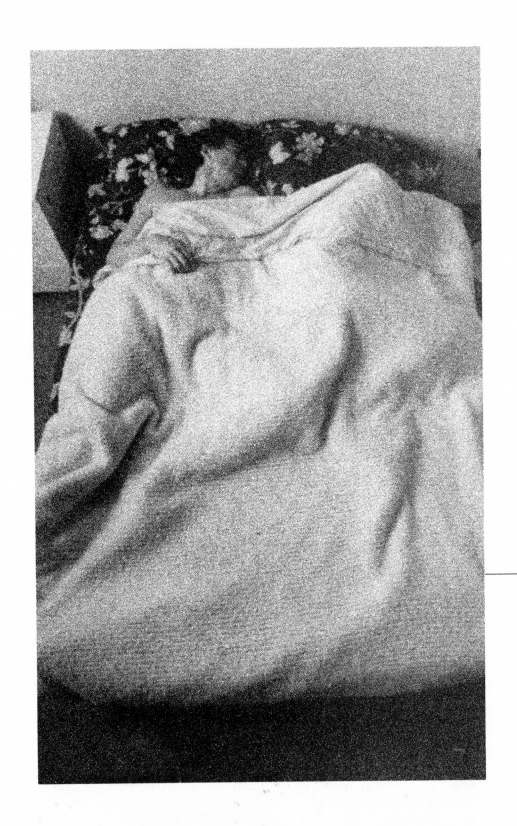

Making It Through the Night

CHAPTER 11

Understanding Sleep Problems

A sleep problem is not "in your head," or for that matter, in your body—but in both. Sleep reflects how you feel, physically and emotionally. Your sleep may be more sensitive to problems of mind or body than your waking consciousness. Throughout the day you may cope marvelously with the challenges and stresses of life. You carry on despite a headache or pulled muscle, frustration, or sadness. Yet however competent you are by day, you can't rely on the same coping skills by night. The signals of mind and body about minor pains or unspoken fears can be ignored during the day, but at night they insist on acknowledgement. Your will, the mainstay of your daytime effectiveness, works against you when you order yourself to sleep. The more you try to sleep, the more wide-awake you feel. If you awaken in the night, you may feel uneasy and vulnerable in the darkness. If you wake up too early in the morning, you may feel grim and isolated waiting for the dawn. If you are drowsy through the day, you may feel less confident and competent.

It is important to recognize what a sleep problem does both to the mind and the body. Such self-understanding begins with self-knowledge. You may be surprised to find out how much you *don't* know about how—and how well—you sleep. To deepen your understanding of your nights, you have to do some homework. This chapter provides questionnaires and guidelines to help you determine what really goes on when you lay yourself down to sleep.

But you have to keep the objective parameters of sleep in perspective. A good night's sleep is not necessarily the same as eight hours spent horizontally.

What really matters is how you perceive and respond to the way you sleep. The key to understanding sleep problems is to learn about yourself, as well as the problem you have.

What insomnia is—and isn't

Insomnia is a misused and overused term that is applied to a multitude of sleep problems. The assumption is that all forms and causes of sleeplessness are the same; therefore, they are all cases of insomnia (which translates literally into "not sleep"). But there is a fundamental misunderstanding in this assumption. Insomnia is *not* a disease, like diabetes or pneumonia, but a symptom, like a fever or runny nose. Focusing only on a symptom isn't likely to solve the underlying problem. But this is exactly what many people who have sleep disorders try to do.

The term "insomnia" is too vague to be helpful, even when used to describe the effects rather than the cause of a problem. For years, sleep researchers have struggled to develop a specific, practical definition. One suggestion was to list the following criteria for "insomnia":

- inability to fall asleep within thirty to forty-five minutes
- reduced total sleep (less than six hours)
- nighttime awakenings that add up to thirty to sixty minutes or more
- excessive daytime tiredness
- subjective complaints of poor sleep

But when these guidelines were used in evaluating 122 people who complained of poor sleep, only 11 of them met at least three of the criteria. The patients' problems were real enough, but the definition proved to be inadequate. Because "insomnia" represents such a spectrum of complaints, it is used in most sleep centers, and in this book, only in its broadest sense.

While only a small proportion of people think they have "insomnia," many more report that they have specific sleep difficulties. When Stanford University researchers conducted a telephone survey of people in the San Francisco Bay Area, only 4.3 percent said they were insomniacs, but more than 38 percent said they had one of the following sleep difficulties:

- problems falling asleep
- problems getting back to sleep after awakening during the night
- awakening too early in the morning
- daytime tiredness caused by nighttime sleepiness.

Telling time in the dark

"I didn't sleep a wink last night." This is a familiar refrain of people who have sleep problems; but it's an exaggeration. What's surprising is how much of an exaggeration your estimate of sleeplessness may be.

Sleep researchers have found that most people aren't good at estimating time during the night. People with sleep problems are particularly inaccurate in judging how much time they spend awake and asleep in a night. In one study, 81 percent of normal sleepers were able to estimate accurately, within ten minutes of the actual time, how long they took to fall asleep, but only 25 percent of the troubled sleepers could. More than half of the insomniacs misjudged their sleep latency time by twenty-five minutes or more. When asked about their total sleep time, 70 percent of the normal sleepers—but only 35 percent of insomniacs—guessed within fifteen minutes of the actual total. Half of the insomniacs underestimated their time asleep by sixty minutes.

Researchers have verified such discrepancies again and again in sleep laboratories. Generally the more severe an actual sleep disorder, the more exaggerated the sleeper's claims about nighttime rest and wakefulness. Sometimes the objective data of sleep recordings reveal that, despite subjective complaints about sleep, sleep times are normal or even longer than normal. Is such "pseudoinsomnia" a form of hypochondria? Many researchers do not think so. It could be that these poor sleepers have abnormal sleep patterns that are too subtle for current monitoring equipment to pick up. In a number of such patients, researchers have found unusual variations, such as different types of brain waves or increased levels of brain chemicals; they don't yet know how to interpret these discrepancies. Whatever the underlying cause of the complaints, there is no question that "pseudoinsomniacs" are just as dissatisfied with their sleep as those whose symptoms are verified by all-night recordings.

How sleep problems start

Jane goes to bed at 11:00 P.M. each night, falls asleep around 11:30 P.M. and gets up at 6:30 A.M. Joan also goes to bed at 11:00 P.M., falls asleep around midnight and wakes up at 7:30 A.M. Which woman has the sleep problem? Joan—even though she spends an hour more in bed and a half hour more asleep, she is unable to fall asleep quickly.

This tale of two women illustrates a critical point: a sleep problem is not a matter of quantity of sleep but of quality. You may sleep 8½ hours a night and wake up tired and yawn through the day. Or you may sleep 5 hours a night and have no complaints at all. More is not better when it comes to sleep. What matters most is how you feel the next day. A good night's sleep is what amount of rest makes you feel refreshed in the morning.

People do not suddenly "come down with" a sleep problem one night in bed. Sometimes a traumatic daytime event triggers a sleep disturbance. Sometimes the difficulty develops gradually as a result of bad habits or irregular schedules. Tracing the history of your sleep complaint can provide important clues that may point to a possible cure. A sleep specialist was able to track one woman's sleep problems to the time of her marriage: it wasn't her relationship with her husband that was keeping her up nights but the powerful hormones in the birth control pills she had begun to use. Others have looked back at the nights of their lives to discover that their sleep complaints coincided with the start of a new work shift, a return to school, or the seasonal flare-up of pollen allergies.

Researchers have also found that a larger-than-expected number of poor sleepers developed their problem in childhood or adolescence. These lifelong insomniacs seem to have an organic (physical) predisposition to sleep problems, according to sleep researcher Ernest Hartmann, M.D. Of the 100 patients with serious sleeplessness that he studied, 33 had trouble sleeping as children and had been told by parents that they were poor sleepers. While their first sleep complaints may have occurred during a period of acute depression, they did not suffer from chronic depression. Sometimes a trauma, such as an auto accident or a frightening drug experience, caused the initial problem. Most of these people, however, experienced gradual onset of sleeplessness, with more problems in periods of tension, stress, or depression. Disturbed sleep usually did

Making It Through the Night

not lead to medical complaints until the insomniacs were in their twenties or thirties. As adults, they became so fatigued that they found it difficult or impossible to work. Psychological tests showed relatively little emotional imbalance; the most typical finding was a severe and unusual reaction to even minor amounts of psychoactive drugs. Some researchers believe that patients with childhood-onset insomnia, who often have the most intractable sleep problems, may have undetected abnormalities in the systems that control wakefulness and sleep.

The psychology of sleep problems

Troubled people have troubled sleep. This is the most obvious correlation that researchers have found when they looked at the connections between sleep and emotional well-being. Virtually all patients with severe depression report sleep difficulty; most of those with lesser degrees of anxiety and depression complain about sleep.

Is this a causal association? Is poor sleep the result of psychological disturbance? Is it a sign of emotional upheaval or psychic conflict? There are no sure answers. When sleep researchers at the University of Cincinnati administered psychological tests to people with sleep problems and normal sleepers, they found differences in only one aspect of personality and behavior: a condition called "psychasthenia," which is characterized by anxiety and obsessive worrying. The insomniacs themselves attributed their sleep disturbances to worries about personal adjustment problems and the study confirmed their self-observations.

Another psychological trait seems to characterize many people with chronic sleep problems: a sense of hopelessness and helplessness. Insomniacs believe that nothing can help them sleep better. This attitude turns into a self-fulfilling prophecy. When psychologists have worked with patients on specific behavioral remedies for sleep problems, they found this sense of futility to be one of the most common and difficult barriers to overcome. Even when such patients realize intellectually that a sleeping pill will not help, they continue taking pills and argue that nothing else will work. They don't recognize their dependency on drugs, and they feel totally incapable of helping themselves sleep better.

This self-defeating attitude can be overcome. When chronic insomniacs find a way of improving sleep even slightly, they usually start sleeping better rather quickly. The reason? A renewed sense of confidence and control.

Any therapy for a medical problem is likely to help 30 percent of the patients feel better. The reason for this is the "placebo" effect. A placebo (from the Latin for "I will please") has no healing properties in itself. It works because the user believes it will work. In some cases, the patient's belief is so strong that placebos can relieve pain as effectively as a standard analgesic. Any technique or tablet used for better sleep is bound to have a similar effect. For your own sake, and for the sake of your sleep, you'll be far better off believing in your own ability to sleep better than in the powers of a pill (see "The Perils of Sleeping Pills," page 129).

Your "typical" night's sleep: a self-portrait

You probably know most of your vital statistics: height, weight, age, blood pressure, perhaps even your resting heart rate or cholesterol level. You might also think you know your nighttime vital signs: usual bedtimes and wake-times, time needed to fall asleep, number of awakenings, time awake in the night, total sleep time in a twenty-four-hour period. But have you actually documented any of these nocturnal variables? Or are you guessing? In order to help yourself sleep better, you need to be sure you understand how you sleep now. The following questionnaires are designed to help you to understand how long and how well you sleep and to identify any sleep problems you may have.

How you see your sleep

Before you do anything else, fill out the following questionnaire; it will serve to illustrate the way you *think* you sleep. Reflect back on the nights of the past two weeks, and base your answers on your memory of those nights. This may seem like an easy, obvious exercise. However, when you compare these answers to those you give after you start making nightly observations, you may be surprised.

1 ◆ Are you usually sleepy at bedtime? ☐ Yes, very ☐ Moderately ☐ No, not at all

2 ◆ Do you usually follow a sleep ritual before getting into bed? ☐ Yes, always ☐ Usually ☐ Rarely ☐ Never

3 ◆ Rate your typical bedtime mood on a scale of 1 to 10:

1	2	3	4	5	6	7	8	9	10
Anxious				*Tense*				*Relaxed*	

4 ◆ What time do you usually go to bed?

5 ◆ Is this a regular bedtime? If not, what is your typical weekday bedtime? typical weekend bedtime?

6 ◆ How long does it take you to fall asleep? On weekdays? On weekends?

7 ◆ Do you awaken in the night? How often? How long?

8 ◆ What do you do when you wake up in the night or too early in the morning?

9 ◆ What time do you usually wake up?

10 ◆ What time do you get out of bed? Weekdays? Weekends?

11 ◆ Rate your typical morning mood on a scale of 1 to 10.

1	2	3	4	5	6	7	8	9	10
Extremely sleepy				*Groggy, sluggish*				*Alert, energetic*	

12 ◆ Do you feel extremely sleepy during the day? Any particular time of day?

13 ◆ Do you nap during the day? How often? For how long?

14 ◆ How many hours do you typically spend sleeping in a twenty-four-hour period?

15 ◆ Are you dissatisfied with how long or how well you sleep?

16 ◆ When was the last time you think you slept satisfactorily?

17 ◆ Do you use sleeping pills? ☐ Never ☐ Regularly ☐ Occasionally

18 ◆ Do you use large amounts of stimulants (coffee, cigarettes, tea, or drugs)?

19 ◆ Do you take any medications regularly?

20 ◆ What do you think may be the cause of any sleep problems you have?

Background data

Only a physician can evaluate your general health and diagnose any specific problems that may be interfering with your sleep. The following questions may make you more aware of symptoms or conditions that could be the underlying cause of a sleep problem. Be sure to bring these to the attention of your doctor or sleep specialist.

The state of your body

1 ◆ Are you generally in good health?

2 ◆ Are you overweight? If so, by how much?

3 ◆ Do you have any chronic medical problems (high blood pressure, diabetes, or others)?

4 ◆ Do you take any medications for these conditions? List name of drug, dosage, and times of administration.

5 ◆ When was your last complete physical examination?

6 ◆ Were there any unusual findings?

7 ◆ List all the major illnesses and injuries of your life, including the dates of onset and recovery times.

8 ◆ Have any of these problems led to lingering symptoms? If so, what?

9 ◆ Do you have any allergies that you know of? Do you have any symptoms—such as respiratory difficulties—that become worse in different seasons?

10 ◆ Do you exercise regularly? How and when?

11 ◆ List any health problems, however minor, that you have had in the past three months.

12 ◆ List all drugs, prescription and nonprescription, that you have taken in the last month.

13 ◆ Is your breathing during the day particularly loud or difficult?

14 ◆ Have you ever felt chronically fatigued?

15 ◆ Do you feel dizzy or nauseated in the morning but improve during the day?

The state of your mind

1 ◆ Have any of the following stressful events occurred to you in the past year? Death of spouse; divorce or marital separation; jail term; death of close family member; personal injury or illness; marriage; fired from job; reconciliation with mate after separation; retirement; family illness.

2 ♦ Are you a worrier? If so, what do you worry about? Are there certain times when you worry most?

3 ♦ Are you impatient?

4 ♦ Are you competitive and/or aggressive?

5 ♦ Do you get depressed? ☐ Rarely ☐ Occasionally ☐ Often

6 ♦ Do you lose interest in other people and things and withdraw into yourself?

7 ♦ Do you get angry? ☐ Rarely ☐ Occasionally ☐ Often

How do you express your anger?

8 ♦ Are you compulsive about your house, work, or studies?

9 ♦ Do you take problems from your job home with you? Do you take them to bed with you?

10 ♦ Do you tend to ruminate over things that have happened to you?

11 ♦ Do you anticipate problems before they arise?

12 ♦ How do you respond to pressure?

13 ♦ Do you cry? ☐ Rarely ☐ Occasionally ☐ Often

How else do you express sadness?

14 ♦ Do you have trouble letting go and relaxing?

15 ♦ Do you take vacations?

16 ♦ Do you confide in many people ☐ , a few close friends ☐ , your spouse ☐ , no one ☐ .

17 ♦ Do you get upset easily? By what?

18 ♦ Do you argue with your spouse or other family members? When?

19 ♦ Do you believe you acknowledge problems in your life and deal with them directly? Or do you tend to pretend things are going well even when they are not to avoid any conflict?

20 ♦ Have you ever seen a psychiatrist or other mental health professional? If so, when? Why? For how long? Why did you stop? Are you currently seeing someone for counseling or therapy? Are you taking any drugs because of a psychiatric problem?

The state of your sleep

1 ♦ How quiet is your bedroom? If it is noisy, what is the source of the noise? What do you do to overcome the noise?

2 ♦ How dark is your bedroom at night and in the morning? Are you ever

awakened by the light? Do you ever need to sleep during the day because of your schedule?

3 ◆ Does your bedroom seem too hot or cold in the night? Do you wake up frequently either to throw off or add a blanket?

4 ◆ Is your mattress comfortable—firm, smooth?

5 ◆ Do you sleep alone?

6 ◆ How big is your bed? Do you feel crowded in it?

7 ◆ What position do you fall asleep in and wake up in?

8 ◆ Have you ever awakened because of your bedmate's snores? Movements? Kicks?

9 ◆ Do you feel you have a regular sleep-wake schedule? (Verify by comparing to your actual sleep diary.)

10 ◆ Do you ever work in bed? How late? How often?

11 ◆ What do you do to relax before sleep? Warm bath, music, yoga, breathing exercises, reading, other?

12 ◆ Do you ever awaken to care for a child in the night?

13 ◆ Do you ever awaken because you are fearful of a prowler or a fire?

14 ◆ When was the last time you slept well?

15 ◆ What other events in your life coincided with the beginning of your sleep problem?

16 ◆ Do you travel often?

17 ◆ Do you often shift your work schedule?

18 ◆ Do you stay up late or sleep late on certain days of the week?

19 ◆ Does anyone in your family have a sleep problem?

20 ◆ Ask your bed partner or roommate to describe how you sleep.

Your sleep diary

The only way to find out how you really sleep is to observe your nights as well as your days. Set aside a two-week or three-week period that is fairly typical of other weeks in your life. Using the form listed in the appendix (page 295) or a small notebook, answer the questions in your diary at the appropriate times: bedtime, when you wake up, and dinner time. Keep a clock by your bed so you can be as accurate as possible in noting when you turn out the light or wake up in the night. Write in your diary at the very end of your day and first thing in the morning.

Making it through the night

After you have filled out the background questionnaires and have written in your sleep diary for several weeks, you should have a fairly good picture of how you spend your nights. Compare what you know now with what you "knew" when you filled out the first questionnaire, "How You See Your Sleep" (page 160). Even if your guesses and your actual record-keeping do not correlate, you should be more aware of the types of sleep symptoms that are troubling you.

The final section of this book is devoted to specific information on your symptoms and sleep problems, what causes them, and what can be done about them. The sleep problems are categorized according to the five most common complaints:

* problems falling asleep
* problems staying asleep
* problems of waking up
* excessive daytime sleepiness
* occasional sleep problems

Each chapter begins with an introduction and a series of questions related to your sleep. If you answer yes to any of the questions, continue reading in that chapter. The questions about specific causes at the top of each subsection will help you focus on the problem or problems that may be keeping you up at night. There are also special chapters on the sleep problems of children and the elderly.

Learning about your sleep difficulties is the first step to overcoming them. The more you know about sleep in general and about your sleep complaint in particular, the sooner you will sleep better. Advances in sleep science have provided more hope than ever before that you will be able to find a way to sleep more easily through all the nights of your life.

CHAPTER 12

The Edge of Night: Problems Falling Asleep

◆ *If you go to bed at different times on different nights, nap during the day, or eat or exercise in the late evening, see "Bad Sleep Habits," page 168.*

◆ *If your mind is filled with thoughts or worries before sleep, or you fall asleep more easily on vacations, see "Stress and Anxiety," page 171.*

◆ *If you anticipate having problems falling asleep each night, or you sleep better anywhere but in your own bed, see "Conditioned Insomnia," page 174.*

◆ *If you feel crawling sensations in your legs when you lie down to sleep, see "Restless Legs," page 176.*

◆ *If you have problems getting up in the morning, stay up and sleep later on weekends, or have difficulty following a fixed schedule, see "Rhythm Problems," page 180.*

◆ *If you drink coffee, smoke cigarettes, or use drugs with stimulating effects, see "Use of Drugs and Other Stimulants," page 182.*

◆ *If you have been using sleeping pills for several weeks, or you have abruptly stopped taking pills after using them for an extended period of time, see "Tolerance to/Withdrawal from Sleeping Pills," page 185.*

◆   ◆   ◆

T he most common sleep complaint is not being able to turn off the mind and body soon after you turn out the light. Generally, the older you are, the longer you spend in the twilight zone before sleep. Sleep "latency"—the period between bedtime and sleep time—is considered to be long if it extends for more than thirty or forty-five minutes.

Your body quite literally has to shift gears at the edge of night—from control by the arousal, or reticular activating, system to control by the sleep, or hypnagogic system. You can fall asleep only if your arousal mechanisms are turned down low enough for your brain's sleep control centers to start to function.

An overactive arousal system is the cause of most transient problems of falling asleep. If you are excited or anxious about the previous day or the day ahead, the stimulation of these emotions will keep you awake. In people with chronic sleep complaints, the problem seems to lie within the sleep system. Even when they are relaxed, their brains do not send out the appropriate signals. The use of drugs—stimulants or sleeping pills—can compound the problem.

If you are searching for a shortcut to sleep, the following questions will direct you to information on specific sleep disorders:

BAD SLEEP HABITS

- *Do you go to bed and get up at different hours on most days?*
- *Do you nap during the day?*
- *Do you exercise late in the day?*
- *Do you eat a heavy meal or large snack shortly before bedtime?*

You can be your sleep's worst enemy. Daytime habits may be catching up with you at bedtime and making it difficult for you to fall alseep. As long as you can sleep when you choose for as long as you choose, you may not experience any difficulties. But when you try to adjust to a job or lifestyle that requires fixed hours, you will have problems getting to sleep. Many people do not see the connection between the way they live by day and the way they sleep by night. Yet most poor sleepers have very poor sleep habits. Sometimes bad habits are the primary cause of the sleep problem; sometimes they add to it.

What causes the problem

Your body craves regularity, and the sleep-wake cycle is one of its strongest rhythms. Constantly shifting your sleep time is like traveling over several time zones by jet. In effect, you create a case of perpetual jet lag without even leaving your home. Long daytime naps, particularly in the afternoon, also interfere with your sleep cycle. Instead of consolidating your sleep into one long period, you fragment it into short periods of less restful sleep.

What you eat, drink, inhale, or swallow affects how you sleep. All substances that act on the brain—including many drugs, nicotine, caffeine, and alcohol—affect your sleep patterns (see page 219 on alcohol and sleep and page 182 on stimulants and sleep). These substances stay in the body for several hours. If you drink coffee at 8:00 P.M., it is still in your body at midnight. If you smoke heavily after dinner, the nicotine also lingers.

A stomach that's either too full or empty can keep you awake. Heavy meals may make you drowsy but tend to interfere with sleep. An empty stomach can be just as disturbing. Too much or too little of another good thing—exercise can also keep you awake. If you spend your days *off* your feet and get little or no exercise, you're more likely to sleep poorly. But if you exercise vigorously several hours before you go to bed, you'll raise your heart and respiration rates. Your body will be ready for action, not rest.

Young people who are making the transition from adolescence to independent adulthood tend to develop both bad sleep habits and sleep problems. Many college students schedule their classes for late morning or afternoon, stay up late each night and sleep in during the morning. A few times a month they stay up all night to cram for a test; on weekends they may party all night and sleep the next day. They eat when they are hungry and may experiment with alcohol and drugs. During summer break or after graduation, they enter the nine-to-five world of business. This is when the problems begin. As long as they sleep, eat, and play at erratic hours, they are plagued by problems in getting to bed at a decent hour and getting up and to the office on time.

Sometimes bad habits start when you are traveling extensively, working on a special project, or recovering from an illness. The parents of a newborn may find their normal sleep patterns disrupted for weeks. Politicians in an election campaign, executives launching a new venture, families moving across the country—all are likely to find themselves eating, sleeping, and working at odd hours. These disruptions affect all aspects of your life, including sleep, and they can lead to the sort of irregular habits that create sleep disturbances.

What can be done

Concentrate on making new habits rather than simply breaking old ones. Start with a conscientious sleep diary; it will help you understand your habits in sleeping, eating, working, and worrying. Self-monitoring can be both treatment and cure. In every case, it is a good beginning.

Following some simple sleep guidelines may help overcome a sleep problem. At the very least, these recommendations should speed up your progress toward a good night's sleep.

1 ◆ *Keep regular hours.* Establish a regular wake-up time. Set your alarm for a specific hour of the morning and get up at that time every day, regardless of how long or how little you have slept. Keep a record in your sleep diary (page 164) of the times at which you go to bed. Do not allow yourself any naps in the day. You will begin to see a pattern that indicates what your best sleep time is.

2 ◆ *Remember that less is more.* You are better off underestimating your sleep needs than overestimating them. If you spend too much time in bed, your sleep will become fragmented and light. You'll increase your sleep efficiency by decreasing the time you lie in bed.

3 ◆ *Don't go to bed too full or too hungry.* If you eat a heavy meal right before your bedtime, you go to bed when your stomach has several hours of work to do. If you must eat dinner late, make it a light meal. Don't make the opposite error, either. It can also be difficult for you to fall asleep when your stomach is empty. If you're dieting, have a low-calorie snack before bed.

4 ◆ *Exercise regularly—but not before bedtime.* Daily exercises help you sleep better and longer (see chapter 3, page 38). However, heavy exercise in the late evening raises your respiration and heart rate and interferes with relaxation. Schedule your work-outs for earlier in the day. Or try some gentle exercises, like stretching or yoga, to help you relax at night.

5 ◆ *Cut down on cigarettes and caffeine.* These stimulants can jangle your nerves

for hours into the night. Individual sensitivity varies greatly, but sleep recordings confirm that these ubiquitous substances definitely affect sleep stages (see page 182).

6 ◆ *Don't drink alcohol after dinner.* Drinking in the late evening may help you go to sleep (or, if you drink enough, into a stupor), but as the alcohol wears off, you may wake up early and restless. A glass or two of wine with dinner is an ideal sleep inducer; a small amount at bedtime also should do your sleep no harm.

7 ◆ *Turn yourself down toward the end of the day.* If you work or do household chores until the time you get into bed, you may feel physically exhausted but unable to sleep. Put your duties aside at least an hour before bed and perform soothing, quiet activities that will help you relax.

8 ◆ *Develop a sleep ritual.* This may be as simple as lying in bed and listening to soft music for a few minutes or it may be a far more elaborate routine that eases you into sleep. Used regularly, it will prove particularly helpful in times of travel or stress.

9 ◆ *Avoid naps.* The more you sleep by day, the more inefficiently you sleep by night. And the longer the nap, the greater the impact it may have on your nighttime rest. If you feel a regular need for a nap in the late afternoon or evening, try adding half an hour to your nighttime sleep.

Try to maintain some semblance of order when circumstances require nonstop work or travel. Eat your meals at the same times you normally do. Try to get some sleep during your usual sleep hours. And return to your schedule as soon as you can. Remember that the worst thing to fear is not sleeping. Some people struggle so hard to sleep and worry so much about sleeplessness that their fear of insomnia keeps them awake. Even if you do have a sleepless night, it may affect you less than a night of drugged sleep. If you avoid naps, you will eventually get tired at your typical bedtime. It is the way of all flesh.

STRESS AND ANXIETY

◆ *Do you sleep much better on vacations and holidays?*
◆ *When you lie down to sleep, do thoughts race through your mind?*
◆ *Could you be described as uptight or tense?*
◆ *Do you like to be in control at all times?*

Stress seems to be the epidemic of the twentieth century, the bane of our high-powered, fast-paced lifestyle. The term "stress" comes from the Latin *stringere*, which means to "draw tight." And this is exactly how we feel when the world is too much with us: uptight, restless, unable to relax. Stress has different effects on different people—by night as well as by day—and it is a common factor in a variety of sleep disorders.

What causes the problem

Sometimes sleep problems linked with tension and anxiety are lumped together under the medical heading of "persistent psychophysiological insomnia." At most sleep centers, a large percentage of patients who complain of sleep problems are also having problems coping with emotional, family, or occupational concerns.

People with sleep problems sleep differently than others. As studies have shown, their muscle activity during sleep is higher; their pulse rates are rapid; their brains produce more alpha waves (which also occur during waking) during the night. They are more easily aroused and wake up more frequently. It may be that some people have more sensitive or more active arousal systems, which fuel them with "nervous energy" during the day and interfere with normal sleep.

GENERAL ANXIETY   When people with sleep complaints are given extensive psychological tests, they tend to score higher than others on various indicators of disturbance. However, even when patients show high anxiety levels, researchers have not been able to prove that anxiety itself is the direct cause of their sleep problem. When their sleep improves, some may still seek psychiatric help. Others learn to manage their anxiety through psychotherapy but continue to have disrupted sleep.

This does not mean that anxiety and sleeplessness are not related. For fifty years the two have been associated, but no one yet knows whether certain people have sleep problems because of anxiety or whether the sleep problems add to the anxiety. Some psychologists have suggested that anxious people tend to "overreact" to external stimuli during the night as well as the day. When studied in sleep laboratories, anxious patients spend more time in the lighter stages of sleep, and some seem particularly sensitive to small changes in the environment. Some studies suggest that they tend to have higher body temperatures and move more at night. Because they worry more than others, they seem to have more difficulty turning their minds off for the night.

HYPERVIGILANCE AND RUMINATIVE INSOMNIA Hypervigilance is a behavior pattern that may be caused by an innately high arousal level. People with this problem usually have characteristic habits during the day: attention to small details, sensitivity to sound and other stimuli, meticulousness, a tendency to mull over any intense experience—good or bad. Even when they are not worried or anxious, they "replay" the events of the previous day or the coming day as they lie in bed. They can keep themselves awake for hours, but sleep normally once they finally fall asleep. A related sleep disorder, "ruminative insomnia," afflicts those who routinely begin problem-solving without anxiety as they lie in bed.

SLEEP PHOBIAS We all have dislikes and fears, and one of the most common is that of being alone in the dark. Fears that grow so intense that they interfere with our daytime behavior or our nighttime sleep are called "phobias."

Some people are afraid of falling asleep. A child may have heard that grandma "went to sleep with the angels" and is afraid of dying. Sometimes people who have frightening dreams are fearful of another night of torment. Soldiers who once had to keep watch through the night may remain wary of falling asleep years after the war. Others may dislike loss of control at any time, night or day, and struggle against weariness. Most people with this problem are unaware of the fear that may make it so difficult for them to relax before bedtime and fall asleep.

Other people have the opposite phobia: they fear that they will develop insomnia and that a sleepless night will trigger a long run of desperate nights. These people may create a sleep problem simply by trying too hard. One pregnant woman, for example, was determined to get more sleep for the sake of her unborn child. She tried staying in bed longer but ended up sleeping less. Her sleep problems kept getting worse as her fears of harming herself and her baby by not sleeping increased. Reassurance and relaxation therapy finally helped her rest.

Anxious people, worried about becoming more tense if they do not sleep, may use—and ultimately abuse—sleeping pills, tranquilizers, and alcohol (see Chapter 10, "The Perils of Sleeping Pills"). These temporary shortcuts invariably lead to less sleep and more problems.

If anxiety is keeping you awake, there are effective coping skills you can learn to use before bedtime. Chapter 9, "Techniques to Help You Sleep Better," provides a variety of relaxation techniques that have proved to work well in turning off an overactive mind. Since no one method has been shown to be superior to the other, you can pick the one that suits you best. The key to success is practicing, so that you are able to induce a profound state of relaxation.

You might also adapt some commonsense measures to your specific sleep problems. If you are a worrier, set aside half an hour or an hour for "worry time" early in the evening. If you are a compulsive planner, use some time in the evening to make up a list of everything that needs to be done the next day. If you try to solve problems from your bed, substitute a long evening walk or a solitary hour by the fire. Quiet and freedom from distractions are what your racing mind needs to calm down.

If you work in the evenings, quit at least an hour before bedtime and perform relaxation exercises or begin a soothing sleep ritual (yoga, a bath, listening to music). One computer programmer went to a sleep center because he kept "debugging" programs when he went to bed. Alcohol, marijuana, and sleeping pills could not turn off the data processing in his mind. Relaxation therapy and an hour of light reading did.

CONDITIONED INSOMNIA

+ *Do you anticipate problems falling asleep even before you get into bed?*
+ *Do you doze off while reading or watching television but become alert when you get into bed?*

◆ *Do you easily fall asleep anywhere but in your own bed—a living room couch, motel room, or camping tent?*

Sleeplessness can be a self-fulfilling prophecy. If you think that you are going to have problems sleeping, you will. If you think you've developed insomnia because of a few nights of lost sleep, you will probably prove yourself right. If you "work" at sleeping better, you will discover that the more you try, the less you sleep. Conditioned insomnia is a sleep problem that gets worse rather than better but mysteriously disappears in any other sleep setting. One man who usually needed two or three hours to fall asleep in his own bed reported that he fell asleep almost instantly on a backpacking trip in a sleeping bag rolled out on a rocky ledge.

What causes the problem

The classic example of conditioning is the story of Pavlov's dogs, which started salivating at the sound of a bell because they associated the sound with feeding time. You may be unconsciously associating your bed with a time or a trauma that is linked in your mind with sleeplessness.

The initial reason you could not sleep may have been a childhood fear, an illness or injury, anxiety about a new job, travel, or the multiple stresses of any life transition. After a few sleepless nights, you started worrying about whether you would be able to fall asleep that night. Perhaps you went to bed earlier— and lay awake longer. Long after the problem that first kept you awake is resolved, you still have difficulty in getting to sleep. Negative conditioning has led you to expect sleep problems, and you make this expectation come true. Sometimes the conditioning agents are external: bed, bedroom, a familiar aroma, part of your routine for getting ready for bed. Sometimes they are internal: an unpleasant association with bedtime from your early childhood, a buried memory about a time of illness or anxiety, anticipation of a phone call in the night.

Conditioned insomnia can persist for years, even decades. Some researchers believe that people who already have some sleep disturbances are more likely to be conditioned into developing more problems. Conditioned insomnia often coexists with anxiety or worry (see page 169).

What can be done

Conditioned insomnia triggered by external cues is rare. However, most people start sleeping better after taking action to cope with even one factor that is disturbing their sleep. Some people run away from their problem and move into the guest room or sleep in the living room. But such diversionary tactics do not always work. The idea is to build up your confidence in your ability to sleep wherever you choose, including your own bed.

If you can identify a single source of anxiety, eliminate it. Firefighters, police officers, physicians, and others who spend some nights on call may be conditioned to lie awake in case the phone rings. Adjusting their schedules so that they know exactly which nights they might be called allows them to sleep better on the other nights. If you get late night calls that are not emergencies, invest in an answering machine or contact an answering service. You will get the message and a good night's sleep.

Perhaps the most effective approach to conditioned insomnia is a strict deprogramming method designed by behavior therapist Richard Bootzin of Northwestern University. This "stimulus control" regimen requires that you stay out of your bed unless you're ready to sleep (see page 120 for detailed guidelines). Stimulus control demands patience and perseverance. You should be prepared for some sleepless or near-sleepless nights. However, researchers believe that this approach can help a majority of the patients who have conditioned insomnia.

RESTLESS LEGS

* *Do you feel creeping sensations in your legs when you lie down to sleep?*
* *Does this intense discomfort force you to move your legs or get out of bed and walk?*
* *Do the attacks recur several times before you fall asleep?*

In the seventeenth century a British neurologist wrote of patients' complaints of "leapings and contractions of the tendon" when they attempted to sleep. "So great the Restlessness and Tossings of their Members ensue that the diseased are no more able to sleep than if they were in a Place of greatest Torture," he noted.

Restless legs are a common problem. However, many victims feel that their symptoms are so bizarre that they must be unique. They complain of problems falling asleep but hesitate to describe the peculiar sensations in their extremities.

What causes the problem

A creeping or crawling feeling usually occurs in the lower leg, between the knee and ankle. This strange sensation may spread to the thigh, the feet, and the arms. Usually both legs are affected, and the feeling is centered deep within the muscles or, as patients describe it, "in the bones." Some victims say they feel as if their legs "are full of small worms" or that "ants are running up and down in my bones."

During the day the discomfort may disappear entirely or occur only if the person has to sit still for any length of time, particularly in the evening. The more bored, quiet, or tired a person is, the more susceptible he or she may be. Some people say that the restlessness bothers them most in boring situations. Others complain they cannot sit through even the most fascinating plays, lectures, or movies and must wander "like lost souls" to relieve the aches in their legs.

The feelings of creeping or pulling intensify at bedtime, usually five to thirty minutes after the person gets into bed. In mild cases the symptoms soon disappear, but they can last for hours. In severe cases they persist intermittently until early morning, so the victim sleeps only a few hours. Usually it is impossible to keep restless legs still. Kicking or moving the legs or massaging them may help. Often the victims have to walk to ease the feeling. One older woman dances the Charleston in her bedroom until her legs feel better. Others pace through their homes night after night. "I feel like Marlow's ghost in *A Christmas Carol*," said one weary wanderer. Even when they fall asleep, many victims of restless legs are awakened by spontaneous leg jerks: more often they awaken their bedmates with their kicks and twitches (for discussion on nocturnal myoclonus, see page 199).

All-night evaluations in sleep laboratories have confirmed how little and how poorly these people sleep. In one case, researchers at the National Institute of Mental Health found great variations in the sleep pattern of a woman with severe restless-leg syndrome. They also found signs of a disease of the spinal nerve cells, as indicated by abnormalities in the woman's record of muscle activity, a biopsy of muscle tissue, and evaluation of her spinal fluid.

Approximately one third of the cases of restless-leg syndrome are inherited. The syndrome is also associated with diseases of the blood vessels, polio, diabetes, anemia, and disorders of the vertebral discs. Sleep deprivation makes the condition worse; for unknown reasons, fever diminishes the symptoms.

Poor blood circulation may cause or aggravate the problem in some people. Pregnant women are particularly vulnerable to developing restless-leg syndrome. In one study, 11 percent of the women developed restless legs in the second half of their pregnancies; the symptoms disappeared after delivery. Restless-leg syndrome becomes more severe with age in some people, perhaps because circulation is often impaired.

What can be done

Sleep researchers are just beginning to unravel the mysterious causes of this unusual problem. They already know that sleeping pills do *not* work. If you cannot get to sleep because of restless legs, consult your doctor or a sleep center. Because this is a very specific complaint related directly to sleep, the specialists at the sleep-disorder centers have greater expertise in recognizing and dealing with it.

The condition of some people improves when they are given drugs that dilate (expand) the blood vessels and improve their circulation. However, these are powerful agents with worrisome side-effects. It is essential for you to work closely with your doctor so you can understand and balance the risks and possible benefits of such medications.

One researcher, Elmar Lutz, M.D., chairman of neuropsychiatry at St. Mary's hospital in Passaic, New Jersey, believes that caffeine may be involved in the development or exacerbation of restless legs, perhaps because it increases the activity of the nervous system. He has reported cases in which young adults developed the syndrome after they first began drinking coffee or large amounts of cola drinks, which also contain high levels of caffeine.

RHYTHM PROBLEMS: DELAYED SLEEP ONSET

- *Do you lie awake for hours after getting into bed?*
- *Do you have problems getting up in the morning?*
- *Do you stay up later and sleep later on weekends and vacations?*

Many people with this problem think of themselves as "night owls" who are full of energy when most others are fading fast. As long as they can stay up all hours and sleep late the next morning, they do fine. But if they try going to bed at a "normal" bedtime of 11:00 P.M. or midnight, they toss and turn for hours. Getting up when the alarm goes off the next morning may be impossible.

What causes the problem

Night owls are different: Their body temperature, which is closely correlated with physical and mental abilities, peaks later in the day. They are coldest—and most lethargic—in the morning and warmest—and most energetic—in the evening. Their sleep disorder is a clockworks problem; they are out of synch with the rest of the world.

This curious biological rhythm may be set in childhood, although it may be innate. Parents tell of one sibling who sneaks a flashlight and books into her bed so she can read while her sister sleeps soundly a few feet away. One twin traced his problem back to early childhood when he stayed up later than his sister so he could have his parents' sole attention.

Sometimes a trauma—an illness, injury, or life crisis—leads to late nights over a long period. Eventually the body will adjust to and insist on the new rhythm. Sometimes this problem is an occupational hazard. Nightclub entertainers may become night people out of necessity, as do others who work a night shift. If sleep time and social and professional obligations are time-coordinated, there is no problem. But when a long-term night owl tries to live a nine-to-five life, there are certain to be problems. Some may feel alienated from family and friends because they still live by a different biological rhythm. Some struggle so hard to get to work on time that they are chronically sleepy. Many try every sleep remedy they hear of, from potions to pills, with no success.

What can be done

The solution to sleep rhythm problems is to reset your biological clock. Researchers have found that it is extremely difficult to try to "phase-advance" sleep times by requiring a person go to bed earlier than usual. Instead they "phase-delay" sleep time, shifting bedtimes later and later until they move the bedtime around the clock to a desirable hour.

Here is how it works: If you normally fall asleep at 3:00 A.M. (regardless of whether you got into bed at midnight or 2:45 A.M.), you move your bedtime forward by three or four hours (different sleep centers favor different schedules). For three or four days you go to bed at 6:00 A.M. and sleep your normal length of time. Then you shift your sleep time forward to 9:00 A.M., stabilize it for a few days, and then start going to sleep at noon. Over a two-week period you can shift your bedtime to where you want it; in this case, to midnight.

"Chronotherapy," as this therapy is called, is effective but demanding. For a one or two-week period, you may be going to bed when others are eating lunch. You will need a place where you can sleep at any hour of the day, and you will need much support and encouragement. It is best for you to work with a sleep specialist in readjusting your body's clock. Some people stay in a sleep laboratory for the entire time; others sleep at home but are carefully monitored by staff members.

For many people, delayed sleep-onset is mild and is a problem only on Mondays or the day after vacation. Each Friday and Saturday night they stay up later. On Sunday they are wide-awake at midnight—and groggy on Monday morning. To prevent these temporary phase shifts, try to keep your weekend schedule closer to your weekday routine. On long vacations, begin shifting back to your normal hours during the final days of your holiday.

RHYTHM PROBLEMS:
LONG OR IRREGULAR RHYTHMS

◆ *Do you get sleepy at different times from night to night?*
◆ *Are there regular time periods when you have extreme difficulty falling asleep at your usual time?*
◆ *Do you have problems adjusting to a fixed schedule?*

Like other timepieces, our internal biological clocks may not always function with the precision we would like. Some people have daily rhythms that are longer than twenty-four hours. Others have irregular rhythms that shift almost daily. Because they must live by the twenty-four-hour schedule of the world around them, these people may have great difficulty in sleeping, waking up, and working in synchrony with others.

What causes the problem

Some researchers believe that in the earliest eras on earth, humans acquired the rhythm of the world around them. This sense of timing led to the organization of sleeping, working, eating, and playing within a twenty-four-hour day. We maintain this schedule because of the time cues around us; the strongest influence is other people.

When people are isolated from others and from any time cues, they lengthen their normal twenty-four-hour cycle, usually to a "free-running" rhythm of twenty-five hours. Some people seem to follow this longer rhythm even though they are not isolated from time cues. People with irregular sleep-wake rhythms may have some days that are twenty-five hours long, some that last twenty-two hours, and some that are as long as twenty-eight hours. Sometimes the cycle is so distorted that it is difficult to discern any difference in activity by day or night. Sleepiness may occur at any time around the clock, and these people may become apprehensive about when and if they will sleep. As anxiety increases, sleep becomes more fragmented. Trying to get more rest, they may spend more time in bed, which does not lead to more time asleep. Daytime naps, chronic use of sleeping pills, and worrying about sleep compound the problem. The cycle becomes more chaotic, and other ills may develop as the body's carefully orchestrated rhythms are shattered.

What can be done

Regularity may not solve the problem, but it can help. Sometimes a period of illness or disability leads to the irregular rhythms. One woman took to her bed for several months after surgery. When she did try to get up, she felt so tired that she continued taking long afternoon naps. Years after the surgery, she was spending twenty-two hours a day in bed, yearning for more sleep and more energy. She rose only to dine with her husband, but resumed other activities from her bed, inviting friends to hold meetings at her bedside. Working with sleep therapists, she gradually restored some semblance of rhythm to her life.

Some people find that their abnormal rhythms are so strong that they cannot adjust to a twenty-four-hour day. Their best solution, since they cannot change their rhythm to suit the world, is to change their world to suit their schedule. One woman, who had been fired from her job because she was unable to get to work on time, became a freelance writer. Others have found jobs in which they could adjust their hours to their internal clockworks.

Monitoring your daily schedule can help you tune in to your rhythms. If you have been using drugs to wake up during the day and go to sleep at night, withdrawal will help restore your natural cycle. Avoid daytime naps. Be careful about timing your meals and exercise. If you get up at a regular time and spend *less* rather than more time in bed, your body clock will start working again.

USE OF STIMULATING DRUGS AND OTHER SUBSTANCES

+ *Do you use any stimulant drugs ("uppers") during the day?*
+ *Do you drink more than ten cups of coffee a day?*
+ *Do you smoke a pack or more of cigarettes a day?*

The "eye-openers" you rely on during the day also can keep you wide-eyed and sleepless at night. Coffee or cigarettes may seem too mundane and ubiquitous to be classified as powerful stimulants, but they are. And like other drugs, they remain in the body long after they are ingested.

What causes the problem

Caffeine is the most widely used stimulant in the country. Coffee is not the only culprit; caffeine is also found in tea, cola drinks (including diet colas), and chocolate. There are enormous variations in the way that different individuals respond to caffeine. Some people seem innately more sensitive to very small amounts than others. Heavy users build up a tolerance for caffeine. Studies have

What's Your Daily Caffeine Consumption?

Coffee   ____ cups   @ ____ mg = ____ mg
(fill in dose from Table 1)

Tea   ____ cups   @ ____ mg = ____ mg
(fill in dose from Table 1)

Cola drinks   ____ cups   @ ____ mg = ____ mg
(fill in dose from Table 2)

OTC Drugs   ____ tablets @ ____ mg = ____ mg
(fill in dose from Table 3)

Other sources   ____ mg
(chocolate 25 mg per bar, cocoa 13 per cup)

         Daily Total   ____ mg

TABLE ONE

Caffeine content of coffee, tea, and cocoa
(*miligrams per serving—average values*)

Coffee, instant	66
Coffee, percolated	110
Coffee, dripolated	146
Teabag—5 minute brew	46
Teabag—1 minute brew	28
Loose tea—5 minute brew	40
Cocoa	13

TABLE TWO

Caffeine content of cola beverages (*miligrams per 12-ounce can*)

Coca Cola	65
Dr. Pepper	61
Mountain Dew	55
Diet Dr. Pepper	54
TAB	49
Pepsi-Cola	43
Diet RC	33
Diet-Rite	32

TABLE THREE

Caffeine Content of Over-the-Counter Drugs (per tablet)

Anacin	32mg
Aqua-ban	100mg
Bivarin	200mg
Caffedrine	200mg
Dristan	16mg
Empirin	32mg
Excedrin	64mg
Midol	32mg
No Doz	100mg
Pre-mens Forte	100mg
Vanquish	33mg

Source: M.L. Bunker and M. McWilliams, "Caffeine Content of Common Beverages," Journal of the American Dietetic Association, *Vol. 74, pp. 28–32, January 1979*

shown that people who drink a lot of coffee throughout the day can drink coffee in the evening and still fall asleep easily. Lighter users may be up half the night after a single cup of coffee with dinner.

Even when people insist that coffee does not disturb their sleep, all-night sleep recordings show that they do sleep differently. In one study of 230 medical students, caffeine prolonged the time they needed to fall asleep and disrupted their normal sleep stages. The spouses who drank more than five cups a day did not report disturbed sleep or increased daytime nervousness. However, they needed their morning coffee in order to feel more alert and at ease. Without it, they went into a mild withdrawal, feeling less alert and more irritable.

The nicotine in cigarettes may be even more powerful. Two recent lab studies at Pennsylvania State University compared fifty adults who had smoked an average of 1.25 packs a day for more than three years with fifty nonsmokers of the same sex and age. There were no differences in other variables, including personality characteristics and use of other drugs, alcohol, and coffee. During four nights in a sleep laboratory, the smokers required fourteen minutes longer to fall asleep, and they were awake nineteen minutes longer during the night. Another study monitored what happened when eight two-pack-a-day smokers quit. Although they were uncomfortable in the daytime, their sleep improved, and the time they were awake decreased 45 percent. The researchers also made an unexpected discovery: the amount of coffee the subjects drank was unrelated to their sleep. The scientists hypothesize that caffeine users develop a tolerance to that drug's stimulation, while smokers do not develop a nicotine tolerance.

The best known stimulating drugs are the amphetamines. They have a dramatic effect on sleep: they delay sleep onset, decrease total sleep time, and sharply reduce REM and deep NREM sleep. As nighttime sleep worsens, users may feel more tired than ever during the day and take ever-larger doses. Overuse of these drugs can lead to a sudden "crash," with sleepiness overcoming the user during the day. Other side-effects of these powerful drugs are anxiety, irritability, personality changes, and problems in concentration; withdrawal can lead to severe depression, with a possible inclination toward suicide. If stimulant users start relying on "downers" or hypnotic drugs to help them sleep, the risks of addiction and dangerous complications increase.

What can be done

The longer stimulating drugs are used and the larger the amounts that are taken, the more difficult the withdrawal will be. Even with caffeine, a relatively mild drug for most people, withdrawal can lead to irritability, depression, and a general sense of ill-being. However, sometimes a few days without caffeine can lead to dramatic improvements in sleep. One sleep center advised a woman psychiatrist with sleep problems to discontinue coffee. She had been in psychoanalysis for several years; she also worked compulsively and lived by an irregular schedule. Even though her other problems remained, her sleep improved when she stopped drinking coffee.

Withdrawal from cigarettes can be difficult and frustrating. A variety of self-help kits and books are available, as well as seminars to help you break the habit. Few people quit cigarettes just for their sleep's sake, but better sleep can be an added benefit for those who stop.

Withdrawal from most drugs with stimulant effects is much more difficult. Check with your doctor if you are taking specific medications because of a medical problem. Explain that you are having problems falling asleep. By lowering the dose, changing the time when you take the drug, or switching to another, similar agent, your doctor may be able to help you sleep better. Never stop taking a prescription drug without consulting your physician.

Beware of taking sleeping pills to counteract the effects of stimulants. You might well become addicted to two different types of drugs. Be aware of how drugs affect you and consider the risks and benefits. Is losing five pounds worth the hazards of taking stimulants? Will you want the extra boost of an upper if you know you will "crash" hours later? If you feel dependent on drugs, seek help from a qualified professional. If you have been taking stimulating drugs for a long time, do not try to quit "cold turkey" or on your own. Do it gradually, with support and supervision.

TOLERANCE TO/WITHDRAWAL FROM SLEEPING PILLS

- *Have you been taking sleeping pills for more than three weeks?*
- *Have you gradually increased the dosages you have been taking?*
- *Have you abruptly stopped taking pills after using them for several weeks?*

Most sleeping pills lose their effectiveness to induce sleep in three to seven nights. The longest-acting one is Dalmane (flurazepam) (see page 137). As sleeping pills lose their effectiveness, users are tempted to take higher doses. This starts a vicious cycle of ever-increasing tolerance and ever-larger amounts. Sudden withdrawal after prolonged use can lead to severe sleeplessness.

What causes the problem

Drugged sleep is not like normal sleep. It is lighter, more likely to be broken by periods of arousal, and has drastically reduced REM or deep NREM stages. (Different drugs have different effects on sleep stages, see chapter 10). Sustained use of sleeping pills may lead to both physical and psychological dependence. The pills that cause the greatest problems of tolerance are: prescription antihistamines, barbiturates, glutethimide, chloral hydrate, methaqualone, ethchlorvynol, and over-the-counter sleep aids that contain antihistamines. Alcohol causes similar problems.

Some people become convinced that they cannot sleep without a pill, even if they are not physically addicted. They may continue to take a sleeping pill nightly for years—regardless of how well or how poorly they have been sleeping.

Other people become convinced that they need sleeping pills after they try quitting. If you are physically "hooked," sudden withdrawal will lead to some very bad nights. You will lie awake for hours, and you may have much more REM sleep than usual. You may have bizarre, frightening nightmares because your REM time, suppressed by the drugs has suddenly been restored. You may also have daytime symptoms of withdrawal (often not until two to four days after you quit), including nausea, muscle tension, aches, restlessness, and nervousness. All these symptoms will pass with time.

What can be done

The best advice is prevention. If you have a sleep problem, think of pills as a temporary option that is best avoided. Never take sleeping pills for a period longer than their proven efficacy. Ask your physician what this time period is or carefully read the label and package inserts.

Making It Through the Night

If you are dependent on sleeping pills, you can quit. But do not do it alone or try doing it "cold turkey." Seek medical help in weaning yourself from pills. Gradual withdrawal can prevent or minimize the more troublesome side-effects of ending your dependency on a drug.

Sleep disorder centers have established protocols for withdrawing patients from sleeping pills: First they stabilize the long-time user with a specific medication taken at a specific time. The drugs are reduced at the rate of one therapeutic dose a week. This slow tapering is continued until all drugs are eliminated. This process cannot be hurried. One sleep center took more than a year to wean a woman from the pills she had relied on for a decade.

Ask your physician what to expect during withdrawal. The long sleep-onset times and bad dreams will not seem as disturbing if you realize that they are a normal part of the process and that eventually you will sleep better. If you have been using sleeping pills for a long time, your recovery may take longer. The after-effects of the drugs may persist for weeks, even months.

Over time your body will return to its natural rhythms. Twenty percent of insomniacs treated at sleep centers are cured once they are withdrawn from sleeping pills. In the majority of cases, the reliance on drugs was masking the true problem. Withdrawal leads to accurate diagnosis and appropriate treatment.

CHAPTER 13

Things That Go Wrong in the Night:
Problems Staying Asleep

♦ If you have been told that you snore, see "Snoring," page 190.

♦ If your sleep is light and fragmented, and you snore or gasp for air during the night, see "Breathing Problems," page 192.

♦ If you have been told that you grind your teeth at night, or you wake up with sore jaws, see "Tooth-grinding," page 195.

♦ If you move your head or body rhythmically at night, see "Rhythmic Body Movements," page 197.

♦ If your bed in the morning looks like you have fought a battle with the bedclothes, or your bedmate complains of being kicked in the night, see "Leg Jerks," page 199.

♦ If you ever wake up in another room of your house with no memory of how you came to be there, see "Sleepwalking," page 200.

♦ If you have been told that you talk, laugh, or cry in your sleep, see "Sleep-Talking," page 202.

♦ If you wake up to find that you have wet the bed, see "Bed-Wetting," page 204.

♦ If you wake up screaming in the night but cannot recall the cause of your anxiety, see "Night Terrors," page 205.

♦ *If you wake up feeling anxious and remember a bad dream, see "Nightmares," page 208.*

♦ *If you have started to wake up often after a period of having nightmares, see "REM-Interruption Insomnia," page 211.*

♦   ♦   ♦

Problems staying asleep are the most varied type of sleep complaints. Sometimes the source of the problem is the bedmate—who snores, for example—and the source of the complaint is the weary bed partner. Sometimes a problem that awakens you or your bedmate in the night is harmless, like sleep-talking; sometimes the things that can go wrong in the night can be life-threatening, like sleep apnea (a breathing stoppage during sleep).

Several of the disorders that occur during sleep seem to be related to one another. Sleepwalking, sleep-talking, bed-wetting, and night terrors are all problems of partial arousal from the deepest sleep stages and are more common in people who spend more than the usual time in Stage 4 of NREM sleep. They also seem to be hereditary, and people with one of these disorders are more likely to have one of the other problems.

While there are no easy or obvious solutions for some of these problems, a greater understanding of why you wake up during the night may help you return to more peaceful sleep.

SNORING

♦ *Does your bed partner or roommate complain about your snoring?*
♦ *Has your snoring ever disturbed people in other rooms or adjacent apartments?*
♦ *Has anyone told you that there are pauses or silences between your snores?*

Snoring is a sound that sets off fury. Snores can alienate neighbors, infuriate roommates, and shatter marriages. Snorers themselves do not even notice the noise, but their bedmates do.

One of every eight people snores, and men are more likely to snore than women. Children under the age of ten may snore, usually because of enlarged tonsils and adenoids. Snoring is less common in adolescence and young adulthood but increases after age thirty. Even the family pet may add to the nightly din, particularly if it is a blunt-faced Boston terrier or boxer.

What causes the problem

Snoring is the result of the blocking of an air passage during sleep. The noise is caused by the vibration of the soft palate as the lungs struggle to obtain a diverted or weakened current of incoming air. The most common causes of prolonged snoring are anatomical: excessive fatty tissue in the throat, large tonsils, nasal deformities (such as a deviated septum). Some behaviors, such as heavy smoking, drinking, or eating before bed, tend to increase snoring. You are more likely to snore when sleeping on your back because your tongue may fall over your throat.

Generally, snoring is only an occasional nuisance, not a serious sleep disorder. However, chronic nightly snoring may be a signal of severe, even fatal health problems. The greatest danger is apnea, a condition in which breathing periodically stops for seconds or even minutes (see pages 192 and 227). The snores of a person with obstructive apnea are distinct: they are louder (some can be heard throughout the house), and they are punctuated with silence. The pause is the period during which breathing is stopped; the gasping, snorting sound marks the resumption of breathing as the sleeper struggles for air. In severe cases, proper treatment is critical: chronic oxygen shortages increase the risk of sudden death during sleep and may cause or aggravate such conditions as high blood pressure and cardiovascular disorders.

What can be done

If you have been told that your snores bellow through the night and are interrupted by odd silences, check with your physician or a sleep disorder center. There may be much more to your problem than meets the ear.

If snoring is only an occasional nuisance, you can try some home remedies. If you stack up pillows to keep your head raised, you will be less likely to snore. Or tie a hard ball around your body or sew it to the back of your pajamas so you will sleep on your side throughout the night.

Sometimes snoring is caused by flabby muscles in the mouth, particularly when dentures are removed. Sleeping with your dentures should eliminate the snoring. Since obesity enhances snoring, losing weight may help you sleep in silence. Allergies may also be the problem. Check with your physician to see if you are sensitive to the materials in your pillow, bed, or bedroom.

Eugene Hinderer, M.D., an ear, nose, and throat specialist at the University of Pittsburgh, recommends a simple preventive technique based on the theory that, as you sleep on one side, the nasal passage on top opens up and the bottom one swells and closes. As you turn over, the reverse happens, assuring quiet breathing through the night. You will snore if there is an abnormality or nasal congestion blocking the upper nostril. Hinderer suggests rolling up a tiny ball of tissue (a piece the size of a postage stamp) and placing it inside the forward pocket of the tip of your nose. If one nostril's pocket is bigger, use a slightly larger piece of tissue. The tissue helps open the nostrils and change the direction of the air current so that the soft palate does not start vibrating.

Most sleep therapists are skeptical of the devices on the market that claim to help you stop snoring. Harnesses that are used to prevent you from turning over may be so uncomfortable that they interfere with sleep. Loud snorers can sleep—and snore—right through snore alarms. And straps that prevent snoring by keeping the mouth shut can impede the oxygen supply to the brain. The only gadget that may work is a pair of ear plugs—for your bedmate.

BREATHING PROBLEMS (CENTRAL SLEEP APNEA)

- *Do you fall asleep quickly but sleep lightly and fitfully?*
- *Does your bed partner say that you snore or gasp for air as you sleep?*
- *Are you sleepy during the day?*

Apnea, translated from the Greek words meaning "no" and "breath," is exactly that: the absence of breathing for a brief period. There are several types of apnea that occur during sleep:

Central Sleep Apnea is a breathing problem caused when the brain fails to send impulses through the nervous system to the diaphragm to maintain respiration.

Obstructive Sleep Apnea is a disorder in which the diaphragm continues to function, but an obstruction of the upper airway blocks the flow of incoming air.

Mixed Sleep Apnea is a combination of the two types.

The symptoms of central and obstructive sleep apnea are often different, although they can overlap. Individuals with central sleep apnea are more likely to complain of very light or fragmented sleep during the night. Although they become sleepy during the day, they are not as overwhelmingly tired as those with obstructive apnea. (This section deals only with central sleep apnea. A complete discussion of obstructive sleep apnea is in chapter 15, page 227.) Sometimes central sleep apnea is the unsuspected cause of sexual problems, and male victims report a loss of sexual drive (libido) and difficulty in having erections. There also is a high correlation with depression.

What causes the problem

The problem in central sleep apnea lies in the respiration control centers in the brain. Since they fail to send the proper messages to the diaphragm, it stops functioning normally and contracts against the closed airway, partially or completely blocking it. Breathing stops for seconds or even minutes until the body signals that oxygen is not reaching the brain. The brain rouses the sleeper—not usually to the point of awakening—who vigorously and noisily sucks in air. These episodes may occur during REM or NREM sleep, but they are longer when accompanied by rapid eye movement. If there is full arousal, the sleeper may recall a sense of choking and a feeling of anxiety.

Central sleep apnea may account for 10 percent of all complaints of insomnia, but its prevalence in the general population is unknown. It seems to be more frequent in persons over age sixty. The overwhelming majority of its victims are males whose daytime breathing is normal. When central apnea occurs before or along with obstructive apnea, the breathing stoppages can be extremely frequent and severe. Sleep recordings have revealed that more than

500 apneic episodes can occur during the night. The continuing interference with oxygen can lead to irregular heart beats (cardiac arrhythmia); if an arrythmia occurs during an apnea, the heart may stop beating. This condition, termed "asystole," can be fatal. Researchers have speculated that sleep apnea, which may affect a large percentage of older men, may be the reason that so many elderly people die quietly and mysteriously in their sleep.

Sometimes central apnea is caused by medical problems, including polio, brain tumors, damage to the brain stem, or severance of the spinal cord. It also seems related to the development of the central nervous system. Some researchers believe that sleep apnea is common in infants under three months of age and is particularly dangerous in premature babies (see page 260 for information on Sudden Infant Death Syndrome). Older children who have breathing problems usually have obstructive apnea, caused by enlarged tonsils and adenoids.

Another breathing disorder, similar to central sleep apnea but extremely rare, is primary alveolar hypoventilation, also known as "Ondine's curse." Unlike apnea, this disorder impairs respiration during the day as well as at night. The central nervous system fails to respond to normal chemical controls for breathing, and there is insufficient ventilation or flow of oxygen through the tiny air sacs (alveoli) of the lungs. The problem is aggravated during sleep, particularly during REM periods, because of changes in the blood gases, but this is not exclusively a disorder of sleep. The name "Ondine's curse" is a reference to a legendary water goddess (Ondine) who was scorned by a man. In her fury, she placed a curse on him: he could breathe only when he thought of her, and thus he could not sleep and breathe at the same time. Scientists believe that the cause of this baffling disorder, most commonly reported in infants, is a disturbance in the central nervous system. In adults, such conditions as extreme obesity, chronic obstructive pulmonary disease, and other ailments that impair the chest muscles may play a role. There are no effective drugs or surgical treatments; patients with this uncommon problem can be hooked up to mechanical ventilators at night to assure that they get the oxygen they need.

What can be done

Diagnosis of central sleep apnea is the crucial first step. If you sleep fitfully, awaken often, feel sleepy during the day, and snore loudly but with periodic silences between snorts, consult a sleep disorders center. You may be asked to take a nap in the physician's office; a respiratory gauge placed around your chest will detect breathing stoppages. However, the diagnosis is usually confirmed by an all-night recording at a sleep laboratory (chapter 19 describes what to expect during a night at a sleep center). If sleep apnea is suspected, your respiration will be monitored to detect any pauses in your diaphragm movements or your respiration. An "oximeter" on your ear lobe will register any decline in the oxygen content of your blood.

Treatment will depend on how severe the problem is. If you are extremely obese, weight loss may help. Central sleep apnea may persist, but it should be less frequent. Some physicians have tried treatment with drugs, primarily chlorimipramine, an antidepressant, but there are problems with this approach, including eventual tolerance to the drugs. In some cases, a diaphragmatic pacemaker, similar to a heart pacemaker, may be used to stimulate normal breathing through the night.

Never take any sleep-inducing drugs if you have or suspect you have sleep apnea. Sleeping pills, alcohol, and other hypnotic drugs are extremely dangerous because they can aggravate the defects in respiration and interfere with the body's warning signals that rouse the sleeper and force breathing. Failure to respond to these signals can be hazardous or even fatal.

TOOTH-GRINDING (BRUXISM)

- *Does your bed partner complain that you gnash and grind your teeth at night?*
- *Do you wake up with sore jaws?*
- *Has your dentist noticed abnormal wear and tear of your teeth?*

Millions of men, women, and children gnash through the night. They generally are not aware that they are "bruxists" (tooth-grinders), although their dentists and their mates are. Researchers estimate that 5.1 to 21 percent of adults grind their teeth. Dentists say that 20 percent of their patients are bruxists. Even though it is a common problem, there's been relatively little research on bruxism, in part because dentists have thought of it as a psychological disturbance and psychologists have viewed it as a dental problem.

What causes the problem

Thirty years ago the *Journal of Dental Medicine* described bruxism as a "symptom of emotional illness" that might represent "the expression of anger, anxiety, hate, aggression or sadism, which the patient has strongly repressed from his consciousness." Psychologists have suggested that some people grind their teeth to gratify oral pleasure needs denied in childhood. Some say it is a way for easy-going people to work out their frustrations and for domineering types to express anxiety repressed during the day. One study attempted to categorize bruxists into "strain" and "nonstrain" varieties. Nonstrain bruxists grind rather than clench their teeth, do it at night, and may have a genetic predisposition. Strain bruxists are daytime clenchers of teeth and jaws whose habit seems to be a reaction to stress.

Much of the problem may actually be in the mouth rather than in the mind. Missing, elongated, or poorly filled teeth, as well as such minor defects as rough cusp ends, may be the cause. In these cases, restoration of the teeth or adjustment of the fillings eliminates or reduces the habit. Malocclusion, an abnormality in which the upper and lower jaws do not meet well, may be a factor, but not all people with this problem grind their teeth—and not all bruxists have malocclusions.

The earliest medical theories about bruxism postulatd that the fault lies within the brain. Some neurological disorders, such as epilepsy and cerebral palsy, have been linked to bruxism, as have diseases such as allergies, hyperthyroidism, and endocrine imbalances. Mentally retarded children, particularly those with Down's syndrome, have a greater incidence. There also seems to be a genetic predisposition in some patients.

Bruxism may occur in all stages of sleep, but particularly Stage 2 of NREM sleep. It may be a disorder of partial arousal that occurs during a lightening of sleep, such as the transition from deep NREM sleep to lighter stages. It is associated with other physiological changes, including an increased heart rate.

What can be done

If untreated, bruxism can cause serious damage to teeth, the structures around the teeth, the gums, and the muscles of the mouth and jaw. Even if sleepers do not realize that they are grinding their teeth at night, they may feel the daytime consequences, including facial pain and muscle and tooth sensitivity.

If bruxism is caused by poor fillings or other dental problems, go to a dentist. Some dentists recommend that a bite-plate be worn during the night. While this does protect the teeth from excessive wear, it does not eliminate the problem.

One of the most effective therapies is surprisingly simple: a teeth-clenching exercise. Clench your teeth firmly for about five seconds and then relax for five, repeating this exercise four to six times a day. In one study, after ten to twelve days of this self-treatment, 75 percent of the patients stopped grinding their teeth. Sleep researchers also documented the success of teeth-clenching therapy in a twenty-six-year-old college student whose wife complained about the noise of his jaw-clenching at night. He started exercises of tightening and loosening his jaw muscles for alternate periods of one minute, six times a day. Within ten days he stopped grinding his teeth. Six months later he remained completely cured.

Biofeedback (see page 122) has also been helpful for some patients. In one experiment, sleep researchers used an electrical signal that made the sleepers stop bruxing without awakening them. Even when asleep, the patients "learned" to stop their mouth movements. In another study, the United States Army reported that 75 percent of soldiers with bruxism improved after biofeedback training.

Other therapists have used hypnotic suggestions to help bruxists. In one experiment a hypnotist instructed his patients to repeat the phrase, "Lips together, teeth apart" throughout the day. Occasionally a physician will prescribe Valium (diazepam), a minor tranquilizer), for bruxism. However, researchers consider this the treatment that is least likely to succeed.

RHYTHMIC BODY MOVEMENTS

- *Do you move your head or body rhythmically as you fall asleep?*
- *Has your bed partner ever commented on movements that you make in your sleep?*

Human infants and other primates often rock themselves to sleep, particularly if they are alone. In some children, these movements may become violent, including banging of the head (a problem called "jactatio capitis nocturnus") and rolling of the body. Usually these motions have no physical cause, but they seem more common in children with subnormal intelligence. Environmental stresses, such as parental pressure to do well in school, also may play a role. Although the movements generally stop in adolescence, they occasionally continue into adulthood. In rare instances, they may start in adulthood.

What causes the problem

There are few reports on rhythmic motions before or during sleep in adults. Some researchers have suggested that insomniacs may try to rock themselves to sleep. Others think the activity is related to what happens during sleep. Quentin Regestein, M.D., a psychiatrist at Harvard Medical School, has described a healthy young woman who rocked her head vigorously during REM sleep. She never awakened or knew of her activity until her roommate pointed it out. Sleep researcher Ian Oswald of Edinburgh studied rocking "of remarkable vigor" in two males, one of age thirteen and one twenty years old. Their motions, including head and body rolling and head banging, intensified during REM sleep but did not rouse the sleepers. He theorized that the movement was associated with "some form of disquieting mental life present during sleep."

Sleep researchers at Baylor University found another interesting case: a thirty-nine-year-old investment counselor who had been paralyzed since age nineteen. During sleep he rocked rhythmically, often reaching down and rubbing his lower legs for five to twenty minutes at a time. The rocking was always followed by REM sleep; heart rate and respiration were normal throughout. When awakened while rocking, the patient could not recall the motion. When it was described to him, he remarked that it was similar to the exercises he had done to maintain muscle tone after his injury. He had not performed the exercise during the day for more than five years. His case was the first report of sleep-rocking associated with a previously learned conscious behavior.

What can be done

Body movements—even when rigorous—do not seem to disturb the sleeper. Their bedmates might be advised to move to another bed if they cannot sleep because of the activity. There are no "therapies." Since the movements may relieve unhappy thoughts during sleep and comfort the sleeper, they may actually be therapeutic in themselves.

LEG JERKS (NOCTURNAL MYOCLONUS)

* *Does your bed partner complain about being kicked in the night?*
* *Does your bed in the morning look like you have fought—and lost—a battle with the bedclothes?*
* *Are you excessively sleepy during the day and cannot understand why?*

Your sleep problem may be in your legs. Nocturnal myoclonus is characterized by periodic movements, particularly of the lower limbs, during sleep. These repeated leg jerks can awaken the sleeper—or a bedmate—during the night. Because the sleeper is disturbed, even if not fully awakened, nocturnal myoclonus causes sleepless nights and sleepy days. An estimated 15 to 20 percent of complaints of insomnia are caused by jerking legs.

What causes the problem

Each leg jerk may last only five to fifteen seconds, but a series may last for several hours in the night. Some patients have 300 to 400 leg movements a night, occurring as often as every twenty to forty seconds. Generally both legs are involved, but either leg may move with no obvious pattern. These jerks seem independent of body movements during sleep and always involve extension of the big toe, plus partial flexion of the ankle, knee, and sometimes the hip. The contractions begin *during* sleep, unlike restless leg syndrome, which occurs during drowsiness (see page 174). It affects men and women, primarily when they are middle-aged or older. There may be a familial predisposition, but the problem is rare in children. (Patients with restless legs also often have nocturnal myoclonus.) It may be caused by a variety of medical problems, including drug withdrawal, apnea (page 192 and 227), narcolepsy (page 222), metabolic disorders, and kidney disease.

Physicians do not know the precise mechanism that triggers night movements in the legs. Some speculate that the cause may be improper regulation of the REM mechanism that suppresses muscle tone during dreaming; the jerks might be an overreaction to the inhibition. Sleep recordings show that victims have aroused brain wave patterns, with light sleep and frequent awakenings.

What can be done

Since you are unaware of these movements, even though they disturb sleep, there is little you can do on your own to stop leg jerks. This is a problem that you should discuss with a physician, who may want to perform neurological tests to rule out epilepsy or other disorders. Sleep centers are the best places to go for help, and your therapist may request that you spend a night in the lab to verify that the problem is nocturnal myoclonus. Chapter 19 describes what to expect in a sleep laboratory.

Physicians have tried different drugs to treat nocturnal myoclonus. Valium (diazepam), a minor tranquilizer, has been shown to reduce the number of arousals to twenty to forty per night. Some success has been reported with another drug, Clonopin (clonazepam), an anticonvulsant. These medications should be taken only under close supervision by a physician.

SLEEPWALKING (SOMNAMBULISM)

◆ *Do you ever wake up somewhere other than your bed with no memory of how you got there?*
◆ *Has a bed partner or roommate told you that you walk in your sleep?*
◆ *Did you walk in your sleep as a child?*
◆ *Do you have relatives who walk in their sleep?*

Sleepwalkers seem like creatures from another world. They walk at night with eyes open, faces bland, unresponsive to others. Some have compared sleepwalking, or somnambulism, to a hypnotic trance, explaining it as a symptom of neurosis or hysteria. It is quite common in children, and 15 percent of children between age five and twelve walk in their sleep (see chapter 17, page 266). It is much less common in adults.

What causes the problem

Sleep researchers consider sleepwalking to be a disorder of partial arousal consisting of a series of complex behaviors. Usually an episode starts with the sleeper sitting up in bed; often this is all they do. However, some sleepwalkers get up, dress, go to the bathroom, open doors, perform routine chores, swim, or even drive. They may respond with non sequiturs to someone who speaks to them, but sleep-talking is rare. They seem to have some visual ability because they can avoid bumping into objects. However, it is a myth that they can make their way in complete safety. Accidents, including falls down stairways or through windows, can and do happen. Acts of frenzy or violence are quite uncommon, although one woman allegedly murdered her child while sleepwalking—and was acquitted.

Sleepwalking seems to run in families, and males are more likely to take to their feet at night than females. Sleepwalkers may stroll for five to thirty minutes, but they have no memory of their wanderings. Sleepwalking may begin any time after a child learns to walk. Adult sleepwalkers usually remember childhood episodes but did not sleepwalk in adolescence. They return to their old wandering ways in their twenties or thirties.

Sleepwalkers seem to be extraordinarily deep sleepers, and their roaming seems to be related to the processes of deepest sleep. Sleepwalking is preceded by deep delta waves in Stages 3 or 4 of NREM sleep; they give way to a mixture of lighter NREM patterns and brain waves similar to those of arousal. A sleeping child that is lifted to its feet in deep sleep may begin to walk. In children, this abrupt liberation of movement during incomplete arousal seems related to the development of the central nervous system. In adults, it is often linked with a variety of emotional disturbances.

Sleepwalkers have a higher-than-normal incidence of other sleep problems that start in deep NREM sleep, including bed-wetting and night terrors. In adults, fevers, stress, emotional tension, sleep deprivation, and the use of sleeping pills may increase the likelihood of sleepwalking.

What can be done

Adults who leave their beds and wander through the night for periods of longer than ten minutes should consult a physician. Neurological tests are usually performed to determine if epilepsy is causing the problem; sometimes a psychological evaluation is advised. Physicians have prescribed drugs—primarily Valium, a tranquilizer, and imipramine, an antidepressant—with limited success.

Some psychologists have reported that hypnosis can help control sleepwalking. Psychologist Thomas Eliseo of Rockford, Illinois, reported the case of a nineteen-year-old man who was fearful of going away to college because of his sleepwalking. Passive and shy, he found it difficult to express anger or aggression. In the sleepwalking episodes, however, he sometimes glowered like a bear as he stalked through the night. The psychologist theorized that this was his way of being assertive. Through hypnosis, the patient was told not to get out of bed unless he was completely awake. If his feet were to touch the floor, he would wake up. He was told to visualize himself sleeping through the night and was encouraged to assert himself during the day. His sleepwalking gradually ended, ostensibly because of his new sense of mastery and self-confidence.

If someone in your family is a sleepwalker, you should take some precautions: lock windows and doors, block stairways, keep the car keys out of easy reach. If you discover someone sleepwalking, don't waken him or her abruptly. Do nothing unless there is potential danger. If you must awaken a sleepwalker, firmly call his or her name until it reaches through his or her consciousness. Offer reassurances and lead the sleepwalker to bed.

SLEEP-TALKING (SOMNILOQUY)

+ *Have you been told that you talk in your sleep?*
+ *Have you been told that you hum, laugh, or cry while sleeping?*
+ *Do you worry about talking in your sleep?*

You have probably talked in your sleep. But when you do, you are not conscious of it. Sleep-talkers never listen to what they say. And what they say isn't worth staying up to hear.

Sleep-talking (somniloquy) has fascinated researchers, who once hoped to use it as a "window" into the unconscious. Recently, however, sleep researchers have instead found that sleep-talkers do not reveal any secrets—or even make much sense. The sentences heard in sleep laboratories have been brief and mundane. Typical comments were: "You know I had a hard time falling asleep last night," or "I didn't remember what I was reaching for."

What causes the problem

There are two types of sounds made during sleep: sleep speech, in which words are clearly enunciated in an apparent effort to talk, and nonverbal utterances, like laughing and crying. When sleep-talkers are in light sleep, it is difficult to tell if they are awake or asleep. If you talk to them, you will notice less of an attempt to control or censure their thoughts. "Conversation" may be possible in the time that elapses before the sleeper is stimulated into waking up.

You might talk at any stage of sleep, but there is a difference between what you say during NREM and REM sleep. In NREM speech, you talk with little emotion of very mundane things. Only one of every five comments seems related to what the sleeper remembers was on his or her mind. Talking during REM sleep is rare, but comments made during this stage seem more emotional than NREM statements and are related to dream content. In a sleep laboratory, one man said, "Argentina's a long way away." Awakened, he said he had been dreaming of a woman he dated the previous summer who was from Argentina. Another person asked, "What do you think whales eat?" When awakened, he reported dreaming about people on boats who were being chased. People who laugh and cry while sleeping may be responding to scenes in their dreams.

There is no indication that sleep-talking is a sign of psychological or physical disturbance. Scientists hypothesize that the brain may be capable of producing speech via channels that do not involve awareness. Others are looking for a connection to the brain mechanisms that control dreaming.

What can be done

Sleep-talking is not a sleep problem, unless it awakens your bed partner. There is no need to worry about what you say because it is likely to make no sense whatsoever. And if you hear someone talking during sleep, do not expect to hear any secrets. Most likely, you will not even understand what the sleeper is talking about.

BED-WETTING (ENURESIS)

◆ *Have you recently begun to wet the bed again, years after any childhood problems of nighttime bed-wetting?*
◆ *Do you also have incontinence problems during the day?*

Bed-wetting (enuresis) is the most common sleep problem of children (see chapter 17, page 264). By adolescence and young adulthood, the disorder becomes much less frequent. According to U.S. Army studies of young soldiers, 1 to 3 percent of young men of ages seventeen to twenty still have occasional enuresis. Others have reported that 3.6 percent of psychotic patients have episodes of nocturnal incontinence.

What causes the problem

Enuresis is a disorder of partial arousal that occurs in deep NREM sleep, just as the sleeper shifts into lighter sleep. People with this problem tend to be very deep sleepers with a higher-than-normal incidence of other, similar sleep disturbances, such as night terrors and sleepwalking.

Enuresis has a strong hereditary component, perhaps related to late development of bladder control or to congenital malformations. Primary enuresis refers to a condition in which the individual has never had even one period of several months without bed-wetting since infancy. This persistent difficulty may be caused by a lower-than-usual maturation of the central nervous system or of bladder capacity and control. Secondary enuresis refers to a return of bedwetting after successful toilet training.

Adults with enuresis sometimes have a smaller bladder capacity and more frequent and intense spontaneous bladder contractions. In most instances, the cause is a disorder or disease of the urinary and reproductive systems, including malformations; urethral or bladder infection; illness of the kidney, or the metabolic or endocrine systems; and damage to the mother during delivery of a child. Any medical problem that increases urinary output, as diabetes does, may lead to bed-wetting. Enuresis is differentiated from epilepsy, which triggers bowel as well as bladder incontinence.

Like sleepwalkers, people with enuresis have no memory of what occurs. In most cases, they wake up surprised to find the bedclothes wet. In some people, emotional stress may trigger or aggravate problems of bladder control during sleep.

What can be done

If you develop problems staying dry through the night, see a physician. Enuresis can be an early clue to a variety of problems. Your doctor will want to rule out specific disorders, such as epilepsy, infection, diabetes, and sleep apnea (page 192 and page 227). If bed-wetting is associated with a chronic disease the treatment must be aimed at the underlying problem.

Often surgery may be needed to correct an obstruction. Some common reasons for surgical procedures include: ectopic (displaced) ureter in women; a diverticulum (pouch) in the urethra (urine collects in it during the day and is released at night); bladder malformations; or epispadias (the opening of the urethra into a groove on the upper side of the penis or a fissure in the upper wall of the female urethra). Sometimes imipramine, an antidepressant drug which has secondary effects on bladder tone and contractions, is prescribed for temporary use.

NIGHT TERRORS (INCUBUS)

- *Do you wake up screaming in the night?*
- *If you do, do you feel overwhelmingly anxious?*
- *Do you feel unable to move and breathe?*
- *Are you unable to recall what caused this intense fear?*

A night terror is the most intense form of anxiety you can experience. It begins with a piercing scream that rouses the sleeper and everyone else in the house. The victims sit up filled with an agonizing dread, pupils dilated, perspiring profusely, gasping or screaming. Unresponsive and confused, they may have no memory of what terrified them, or they may remember a single, isolated hallucination. While the attack lasts only seconds, victims may remain inconsolable and agitated for several minutes. They often forget the entire incident by morning.

Two-thirds of all adults report at least one such incident in their lives. Six percent report one night terror a week; some people wake up screaming two to four times a week. Children between the ages of six and fifteen are most likely to wake up because of night terrors, which are referred to as "pavor nocturnus" (see page 267). Adult night terrors are categorized as "incubus," a term that originally referred to nighttime possession by a demon or evil spirit. Night terrors seem to be more common in men; the first attack usually occurs between the ages of two and thirty.

What causes the problem

Night terrors, like sleepwalking and bed-wetting, are a disorder of partial arousal. They begin in deep NREM sleep and may be secondary to an abnormality in the developmental process. The actual cause of this problem is unknown. Most children outgrow night terrors by puberty; males, who mature later, continue to experience them longer.

Adult night terrors may be the result of a malfunction in the sleep process. Two-thirds occur in the first NREM period in the night, that is, during the first hour to hour-and-one-half of sleep. They always occur from NREM sleep, usually from Stage 3 or 4. The likelihood and intensity of an attack seems related to the length of the time the sleeper has spent in Stage 4. Apparently, the longer you remain in very deep sleep, the more likely you are to have a night terror. Sleep specialist Milton Kramer suggests that this may be an "opportunity to occur" relationship rather than one of cause and effect. He compares it to the notion that the more miles you drive, the more likely you are to have an accident.

Sometimes a high fever triggers an attack; other physical causes are head injuries and trauma. Fatigue and emotional stress can also precipitate a night terror. In one study, 33 percent of the patients said their night terror started at a time of major life change. About 75 percent said that emotional stress can lead to or intensify night terrors; 15 percent said fatigue had the same effect.

Physiology may be as important as psychology in night terrors. There are some personality differences between people who wake up screaming and people who do not. In one study, 72 percent of night terror victims showed elevated levels of disturbance on psychological tests that assess mood and personality. Some psychiatrists have suggested that emotional conflict may alter the brain's arousal mechanisms, setting off night terrors. One theory is that night terrors are the result of the ego's failure to control normal anxiety.

There is a familial pattern in the development of night terrors. In one survey, 14 percent of the first-degree relatives of victims and 10 percent of their second-degree relatives also had night terror attacks at night. People with other disorders of partial arousal are also more likely to develop night terrors. Researchers estimate that 33 percent of all sleepwalkers and 16 percent of those with enuresis (bed-wetting) suffer from night terrors. As many as 94 percent of people afflicted with night terrors also walk in thier sleep; in some cases, they open windows, fall, injure themselves, or become violent.

The anxiety of a night terror is real and intense. This sense of fear may be produced by the rapid and radical shift in the level of consciousness. The heart rate becomes faster than it ever is by day, jumping from 60 to 80 beats per minute to 170 beats or more. This sudden acceleration may cause the sense of overwhelming dread; the feeling of muscle paralysis may result from intense muscle contraction.

More than three-fourths of adult victims can remember the experience to some degree immediately after an attack. By morning, two-thirds remember the incident, usually only with effort. The quality and extent of recall are limited and may vary considerably.

Unlike nightmares, which rise out of REM sleep, night terrors are not related to complex imagery. Sometimes victims report one simple, frightful scene—most often a chase, attack, or fall. Fear of attack is the most common theme; a chase image produces the highest rise in heart rate; fear of falling is the least common and causes the smallest increase in heart rate.

What can be done

The first step is to build a sense of safety and security in your bedroom. Sometimes simple precautions, like locking windows and leaving on a night-light are reassuring and minimize attacks.

If the attacks are severe and disrupt your rest and that of your family, consult a physician or sleep center. Neurological tests may be performed to rule out epilepsy; generally the results are negative.

The only available therapies involve drugs. Valium (diazepam), a minor tranquilizer, taken in doses of 5 to 20 milligrams before bedtime, can decrease the number of night terrors by decreasing NREM Stage 4 sleep. Imipramine, an antidepressant taken in initial doses of 100 milligrams, has been particularly effective in treating night terrors that occur after concussions and traumatic experiences.

NIGHTMARES (DREAM-ANXIETY ATTACKS)

+ *Do you awaken from sleep with clear recall of a bad dream?*
+ *Did the dream present a clear and credible threat to your survival, security, or self-esteem?*
+ *Do you realize within minutes that a dream awoke you?*
+ *Do you feel shock, fear, or anxiety?*

By their nature, dreams tend to be bizarre and disturbing. A nightmare, or dream-anxiety attack, is like any other dream in many respects, but it is more elaborate, more clearly recalled, and far more unpleasant. Nightmares generally involve more apprehension, misfortune, physical activity, and color—and far less happiness. The intensity and frequency of the nightmares, as well as their ability to disturb sleep, are what make them a sleep disorder.

Nightmares are clearly unlike night terrors. They occur during REM rather than NREM sleep, and victims recall their upsetting dreams clearly, both when they awaken from them and in the morning. The suddenly awakened sleeper feels some anxiety; although there is much less panic and terror, the pulse may be rapid.

Nightmares usually occur during REM periods in the second half of the night. They may also happen during naps that last longer than an hour. Three times as many women as men complain about them, although scientists are unclear whether that's because of biological or experiential factors. The mean age at the onset of troubling dreams is 19.2 years, although nightmares may afflict sleepers from ages 4 to 52. Some nightmare sufferers report three attacks a week.

What causes the problem

Nightmares do not seem to be linked with developmental abnormalities, but there is a familial association. In one study, 20 percent of those with nightmares had relatives who also had frequent bad dreams. Sleepwalkers seem prone to nightmares; 60 percent of those in one group reported frequent dream-anxiety attacks.

In 38 percent of reported cases, psychosocial factors, such as a significant life event, triggered nightmares. Mental stress and fatigue tend to increase the likelihood of a dream-anxiety attack. Some individuals seem more susceptible than others, particularly those with greater-than-normal levels of daytime anxiety. Bad dreams, but not actual nightmares, are a feature of depression. Nightmares increase at times of insecurity, emotional turmoil, anxiety, guilt, and painful or traumatic life events.

In a review of psychiatric reports on nightmares, Milton Kramer found that 50 percent of those with bad dreams recognize recurrent themes. The most common theme is death; others are scenes of being chased, incest, helplessness, and threats of danger. Why are scenes of falling, being attacked, and danger to a loved one so frequent in nightmares? According to some traditional analysts' interpretation, a dream about falling represents fear of a loss of love, occurring most often in a person who was unable to show defiance to a mother who remained independent of her children; the dreamer deals with separation from the mother by substitution and rage. The attack dream may express a fear of castration in men who do not express emotions well and who are protective of their self-esteem. The dreamer's mother may have been deeply involved with her children, receiving much gratification from them; the dreamer deals with separation by defending against the need for attachment. A threat to a loved one is the least common and least frequent theme. Mothers are most likely to be haunted by fears for their children; doctors report dreams that their patients are in danger.

Not all psychiatrists agree with these interpretations or with the notion that nightmare sufferers are more troubled than people who do not have upsetting dreams. Most suggest that nightmares are a sensitive indicator of stress or turmoil in daily life and represent an attempt to deal with anxiety and fear. One controversial theory relates dream anxiety to levels of critical neurochemicals in the brain. Lifelong nightmares, says sleep specialist Ernest

Hartmann, may be an early signal or "marker" of schizophrenia, a severe psychiatric illness. He has studied a small and unusual group of people, plagued by vivid nightmares since childhood, and has concluded that they may have a "certain sensitivity or vulnerability which could be part of a substrate for artistic creativity as well as for schizophrenic illness."

Another frequent cause for nightmares is withdrawal from drugs, including sleeping pills and stimulants that suppress REM sleep. The REM-depression induced by the drugs, leads to intense and vivid dreaming after withdrawal. The first few nights of withdrawal are characterized by REM periods that may last twice as long as usual. The withdrawal dreams tend to be bizarre and extremely frightening, in part because dreams become more intense in longer-than-usual REM periods. The nightmares may so terrify the sleepers that they return to their habit of taking pills or develop REM-interruption insomnia and wake up before they start dreaming (see page 211).

Fevers may increase the likelihood of nightmares. Long periods without sleep (and therefore without dreams) also lead to REM-rebound and longer, more intense, and disturbing dreams.

What can be done

Some people troubled by nightmares seek a way to "drown out" their dreams, either with alcohol or sleeping pills. However, the use of any drug that suppresses REM sleep can lead to problems of REM-rebound and a return of even more frightening dreams.

If your bad dreams seem to represent conflicts and problems in your daytime life, you may want to seek professional counseling so you can begin to resolve the underlying problems causing your anxiety. Dreams have long been considered paths to the unconscious, and you may be able to learn more about yourself from your dreams.

If you have an occasional bad dream, consider it normal. Many dream researchers say that you have just as many—if not more—pleasant dreams, but you remember only the more complex and troubling ones. You are also more likely to recall dreams during times of stress and anxiety than when your life is going well; this is exactly when your nighttime thoughts are likely to reflect the stress of your days.

Dream specialists urge dreamers to use their dreams, bad and good, to resolve problems. Some believe that it may be possible to tinker with your dreams so that they are less frightening. If you have nightmares about being chased, you might teach yourself to dream that you suddenly stop, confront and defeat your attacker or that you sprout wings and fly away. Chapter 4, "The Dreaming Mind," describes the recent reports on creative dreaming and ways of rewriting your "dream scripts."

REM-INTERRUPTION INSOMNIA

- *Do you awaken several times in the night?*
- *Do you recall having nightmares before you began to wake up often at night?*
- *Do you wake up regularly at the same time every night?*

REM-interruption insomnia is not common, but it can be very severe. With this disorder sleepers awaken in the first REM period of the night, about ninety minutes after falling asleep, and continue to waken in at least 75 percent of the subsequent REM periods. Often they cannot fall back to sleep and lose four to six hours of rest each night. Men are more prone to this problem than women, and it becomes more common in both sexes after age thirty-five.

What causes the problem

REM-interruption insomnia seems to be strongly linked to emotional disturbance, particularly depression. Frequently, people with this problem had been having severe nightmares (see page 208); interruptions of the dream periods may have become a learned but unconscious way of avoiding bad dreams. The awakenings, usually lasting for more than several minutes, do not cut down on total REM time, but they do break up REM sleep into shorter periods. Researchers believe that nightmares are more likely to occur in longer REM times.

Sleep laboratory recordings have confirmed that REM-interruption insomnia is a distinctive sleep disorder. The awakenings seem to occur after REM sleep has fully developed and may be related to a sudden burst of rapid eye movements, which may signal the start of a vivid dream.

This syndrome may be particularly likely to occur after a traumatic event that had triggered recurring nightmares. One woman began waking up from nightmares after a suicide attempt by her daughter; several months later she sought help because she could not sleep through the night. Therapists traced her REM-interruption insomnia back to the nightmares and her feelings about her daughter's actions. As she came to terms with her emotional problems, her sleep problems ebbed.

REM-interruption may interfere with psychological well-being as well as with sleep. Sleep researcher Ramon Greenberg, who first described this syndrome in 1967, suggests that REM-interruptions may aggravate other psychological symptoms. When nightmares are eliminated by frequent arousals, psychiatric patients have shown other signs of disturbance, including increased depression and paranoia. When patients were given psychological tests, they showed more impaired functioning after nights of REM-interruption. Interfering with the normal dream cycle seems to interfere with the mind's integration of experience.

What can be done

Drugs that suppress REM sleep seem to be only a temporary way of coping with this problem. The sleeplessness may be a signal that the dreamer needs help in dealing with conflicts or traumatic events. Because the underlying cause of the problem is psychological, sleep will be disturbed until the emotional problems are recognized and treated. If you have had troubling nightmares and now wake up frequently during the night, you should seek professional counseling.

CHAPTER 14

The Mornings After: Problems of Waking Up

◆ *If you have lost your appetite and energy, find it hard to concentrate or remember, or feel isolated and sad, see "Depression," page 214.*

◆ *If you also lie awake for hours after getting into bed, see "Circadian Rhythm Disorders," page 216.*

◆ *If you are unable to move just as you are waking up, see "Sleep Paralysis," page 216.*

◆ *If you are so disoriented in the morning that you cannot function normally, see "Sleep Drunkenness," page 217.*

◆ *If you always wake up feeling unrefreshed, regardless of how long you have slept, see "Nonrestorative Sleep," page 218.*

◆ *If you drink heavily before going to bed, see "Alcohol-Related Problems," page 219.*

◆　　◆　　◆

I f you awaken by dawn's early light long before you want to get out of bed or if you cannot rouse yourself at the sound of your alarm, your problem is one of unfinished sleep. The cause may be depression, a malfunctioning internal time clock, or abnormalities in the systems that control sleep and awaking. Very often problems of awaking occur along with other sleep problems, such as difficulty in falling asleep or frequent awakenings in the night. In order to cope with the mornings after, you need to look into what is going on during the night—and the day—before.

DEPRESSION

◆ Do you usually awaken early in the morning, unable to return to sleep?
◆ Do you have some problems in falling asleep?
◆ Do you feel a loss of energy, appetite, and sexual drive or a sense of isolation or sadness?
◆ Are you finding it hard to concentrate or remember things?

Depression is so ubiquitous in our society that it is described as the "common cold of mental health." Most people suffer depression in the wake of a traumatic event in their lives or during a painful life transition. Most of these depressions, like the common cold, run their course in time.

In its more severe and chronic forms, depression can be a life-threatening illness. While depressed people often feel sad, depression is far more than sadness. A depressed person feels anxious, withdraws from others, is agitated, lacks energy and cannot function normally. Virtually all depressed people have sleep problems, particularly early-morning awakenings.

What causes the problem

Depression is a complex and varied problem that occurs in small children as well as the elderly. Many psychiatrists think that this problem is underdiagnosed in our society because many depressed people do not show obvious signs of sadness. Men, who tend to be unwilling to express their feelings and cry less than women, are less likely to be recognized as depressed.

Depression can affect many physiological functions in subtle ways. Symptoms include loss of appetite and weight, loss of sexual drive, neglect of appearance and hygiene, "palpitations" or flutters of the heart, shortness of breath, poor memory, inability to concentrate, indecisiveness, feelings of guilt, illogical thought processes, and isolation. Some people, particularly adolescents, sleep more when they are depressed. Most adults sleep less. As their depression becomes worse, so does their sleep. A person with severe depression has less total sleep, less deep sleep, and more periods of wakefulness.

Depression has a profound impact on sleep stages. In "normal" sleepers the first REM period begins ninety minutes after bedtime and is relatively brief; REM periods become longer during the second half of the night. Individuals with specific types of depression enter REM within an hour of falling asleep;

their REM periods may be accompanied by intense eye movements. Just when most people are beginning their longest nighttime dreams, depressed people have completed their REM periods and may wake up, unable to fall back asleep.

Psychiatrists are investigating the unusual dream cycles of depressed patients in hopes of learning more about the sleeping brain and about mental illness (see chapter 5, page 591). They are using all-night sleep recordings to confirm the diagnosis of depression and to evaluate whether or not antidepressant drugs are working. The earliest sign that a treatment will help may be a prolonged time period between falling asleep and REM sleep.

What can be done

Depression, like any problem underlying disturbed sleep, must be treated before sleep will improve. Specific sleep therapies—including relaxation exercises as well as pills—will provide no lasting relief. The use of sleeping pills is especially hazardous in depressed patients because they may be used as a means of suicide.

The treatment of depression depends on its type and severity. Psychotherapy is essential in helping improve the patients' relationships and social interactions. Psychiatrists also may prescribe antidepressant medications. The two primary categories of these drugs—tricyclic antidepressants and monoamine oxidase inhibitors—have no effect on "normal" people but can and do help the depressed. It is believed that they increase the amount of certain chemical messengers in the brain. This may be the way in which they improve sleep as well as relieve the other symptoms of depression.

If you feel that you may be depressed, make an appointment to see your family doctor, who may refer you to a psychiatrist, or call a psychiatrist directly. Seeking help is the first step to getting help—and getting better. If you begin taking antidepressants, be sure to ask your doctor when you might expect relief of specific symptoms (these drugs usually do not show any benefits for three to six weeks) and what side-effects to anticipate. Often these drugs are taken in a single daily dose at bedtime. Once the drug proves that it is helpful, a maintenance dose may be prescribed for eight to twelve months, followed by slow weaning. A small proportion of patients continue to take medications indefinitely. For reasons that scientists cannot explain, some depressed people continue to have unusual sleep patterns even after they recover and function normally during the day.

CIRCADIAN RHYTHM DISORDERS

+ *Do you lie awake for hours after getting into bed?*
+ *Do you periodically have extreme difficulty getting out of bed?*
+ *Do you find it almost impossible to get to work or school on time?*

Whenever your body clock falters, you may have problems waking up on time as well as falling asleep when you would like. The cause of the problem may be delayed sleep onset (page 179) or a sleep-wake cycle that is longer than twenty-four hours or extremely irregular (page 180). Chapter 2, "Sunrise, Sunset," explains the theories of biological rhythms that may help you tell your body time.

SLEEP PARALYSIS

+ *Are you ever unable to move just as you are waking up or falling asleep?*
+ *Does this paralysis last for several minutes?*
+ *Do members of your family report similar feelings?*

The experience of being awake but unable to move is frightening. Sleep paralysis occurs most commonly in narcoleptics (see page 222), but it may also afflict otherwise normal, healthy individuals who may never develop any other symptoms of narcolepsy. Sometimes it is accompanied by vivid and bizarre dreamlike images that can add to the horror of being paralyzed. Some victims report waking up with a sensation of bugs crawling over their bodies but being unable to shake them off; others hallucinate that an attacker is approaching but they cannot flee.

What causes the problem

Sleep paralysis runs in families and is a dominant trait which the mother passes on to her children. Researchers have documented sleep paralysis in several

Making It Through the Night

generations of a family, beginning either in childhood or adulthood. It is particularly common among Canadian Eskimos, perhaps because of a genetic tendency or because the Eskimo culture may create psychological problems by requiring repression of anger during the day.

Some sleep researchers believe that sleep paralysis represents an abnormality in the mechanisms for muscle inhibition during REM sleep. Others have identified one form of sleep paralysis, characteristically occurring in adolescent males, that is caused by depletion of potassium, a nutrient that is vital for muscle contraction. Alcohol and high-carbohydrate meals may provoke these paralysis episodes.

What can be done

Realizing what the problem is and that it is only temporary makes sleep paralysis less frightening. There is a simple way to break the grip on your muscles: Since the eyes can usually be moved during sleep paralysis, make vigorous scanning motions, looking up, down, right, and left. Try to blink your eyelids. Then concentrate on moving your facial muscles. Systematically move your concentration to more distant muscles. Often, intense eye movements alone overcome the paralysis.

External stimulation, even the voice or light touch of another person, can rouse you from paralysis. Explain this condition to your bedmate or family members. They can help you gain control over your muscles. Although no other therapies are indicated, you might want to speak to a physician or sleep therapist simply to gain more understanding of sleep paralysis.

SLEEP DRUNKENNESS

- *Do you feel confused and disoriented in the morning?*
- *Does it take several hours before you start functioning normally?*
- *Do you gradually feel better as the day wears on?*

Monday morning awakenings can be difficult for almost everyone. Sleep drunkenness is similar but far more severe and frequent. Regardless of the quantity or quality of nighttime sleep, the transition from sleep to wakefulness is prolonged and exaggerated. Sleep "drunks" can barely manage to get themselves dressed in the morning. Their movements, particularly their gait, are uncoordinated. Their judgment is clouded, and they seem unable to react appropriately to external stimuli. They may ignore a kettle of boiling water or burn the toast in the oven. Or they may act irrationally or impulsively, sometimes committing such crimes as stealing or shoplifting. Usually their motor skills improve before their perception clears and their judgment returns.

What causes the problem

This relatively rare condition seems to involve the arousal mechanisms in the brain. The few reported cases show a preponderance of male victims as well as a familial predisposition. Sleep drunkenness is more likely to occur if a person is forced awake, particularly from deep NREM sleep. Patients sometimes complain of very deep sleep at night, and researchers theorize that they may spend abnormally long periods in Stages 3 and 4 NREM sleep.

Sleep deprivation, physical exertion to the point of exhaustion, and the use of sleeping pills may aggravate the problem. Sudden withdrawal from heavy and habitual use of stimulants, including coffee, may lead to sleep drunkenness. The symptoms generally wear off through the day, but they may recur at intervals later in the day.

What can be done

Little research has been done on sleep drunkenness, and investigators are just beginning to unravel the possible causes and look for treatments. If you suspect that you have this problem, you should be evaluated at a sleep disorders center (see chapter 19).

NONRESTORATIVE SLEEP

- *Do you wake up feeling unrefreshed even after sleeping for seven or eight hours?*
- *Are you a light, restless sleeper?*
- *Have you been taking sleeping pills for a long time?*

Ideally, we wake up refreshed and raring to go. Nonrestorative sleep does not provide any "recharging" of our internal energy. Its victims complain of light and fragmented sleep. They feel weary when they open their eyes in the morning and exhausted throughout the day. Sometimes their muscles are stiff and achy. However, they're not irresistibly sleepy; they can keep their eyes open and function.

What causes the problem

All-night sleep recordings show that nonrestorative sleep is indeed different from normal sleep. In some patients, alpha waves—the brain waves associated with waking—occur during NREM sleep, so that the brain simultaneously shows signs of arousal and sleep. There also tend to be many brief arousals through the night. Sometimes long reliance on sleep medications can lead to this complaint or mask it so a diagnosis cannot be made accurately.

What can be done

Nonrestorative sleep can be identified only by an all-night sleep recording. If this is a chronic problem for you, consult a sleep disorders center. (Chapter 19 explains what happens in a sleep laboratory and how to find one in your area.) If drugs are the cause of your problem, the sleep therapists will help you gradually wean yourself from sleeping pills. If there is no clear reason for this peculiar sleep, your problem may be extremely difficult to overcome.

ALCOHOL-RELATED PROBLEMS

- *Do you drink heavily before going to bed?*
- *Do you rely on alcohol to help you fall asleep?*
- *When you awaken in the early morning, are you unable to get back to sleep?*

Alcohol is the oldest and most popular sleep aid. Some people sip a bit of brandy before bed; others prefer different types of liquor for a regular nightcap. But too much alcohol too late at night may mean problems in the early morning. Drinking can interfere with the REM periods that predominate in the second half of the night.

What causes the problem

The relationship between drinking and sleep is not simple (see chapter 3, page 363), but the incidence of related sleep problems increases with the amount of alcohol drunk. Alcohol may have a direct effect on sleep because it alters the metabolic pathways involved in producing the brain chemicals associated with sleep. It also affects other functions, including the normal processes of the central nervous system and the liver, that in turn may affect sleep. Chronic alcoholism leads to shorter, more fragmented sleep. Even occasional drinking prior to bedtime increases deep NREM sleep in the early night but decreases REM periods. People who have drunk themselves to sleep not only wake up early but may wake up with all the symptoms of a hangover. Early morning awakening is less common when an alcoholic goes on the wagon. However, a rebound of REM periods may cause vivid, frightening nightmares throughout the night.

What can be done

The best advice is preventive: do not try to drink yourself to sleep. The price you will pay will come a few hours later, when you wake up with a pounding head and aching body. Generally alcohol stays in the body for four hours. Wine with dinner may help you relax and will not interfere with your sleep because its effect will wear off by bedtime. A small amount of wine or liquor later in the evening should not disrupt your sleep. But be careful. The morning after the night before can be a miserable one.

CHAPTER 15

Yawns in the Afternoon:
Problems of Excessive Daytime Sleepiness

◆ *If you become irresistibly sleepy during the day, have vivid hallucinations as you wake up or fall asleep, and sometimes lose control of your muscles, see "Narcolepsy," page 222.*

◆ *If you snore raucously, with silences between loud, gasping snorts, and have headaches in the morning, see "Breathing Problems," page 227.*

◆ *If you have a chronic illness or have been taking medications, see "Medical Causes," page 230.*

◆ *If you rely on stimulants (coffee, cigarettes, drugs with stimulating properties) to stay awake, or if you have suddenly stopped using these substances, see "Drug-Related Sleepiness," page 231.*

◆ *If you feel unusually drowsy only in certain weeks or months, see "Periodic Hypersomnias," page 233.*

◆ *If you have problems complying with any fixed schedule or completing complex tasks during the day, see "Other Hypersomnias," page 234.*

◆   ◆   ◆

Sleepiness in the day can be as disconcerting and disabling as sleeplessness in the night; it also may be far more common. We all hit low points during the day; this is a normal part of our body's circadian rhythm (see chapter 2,

"Sunrise, Sunset," page 151). But everyone defines daytime "tiredness" differently. Some people view it as a direct consequence of poor sleep; others feel weary even when they sleep long and well. Sleep researcher Ernest Hartmann, in his theory of a "psychology of tiredness," distinguishes between the physical fatigue you feel after a long hike or strenuous exertion and the mental fatigue you experience after a stressful day at work. In the long run, psychological wear-and-tear takes more of a toll on daytime energy and nighttime rest.

Sometimes tiredness masks another problem, such as boredom, poor nutrition, frustration, depression, or drug overuse. Underexertion can be more tiring than overactivity because the body does not get the opportunity to rid itself of waste substances and restore energy and fuel to the muscles. Daytime sleepiness is more of a problem for the sedentary than for hard laborers or athletes.

Sleepy people often are dismissed as lazy or less than bright. However, sleep researchers have found many strong reasons to regard complaints of yawns in the middle of the day very seriously. This chapter discusses the variety of sleep disorders—some discovered only recently—that could be the cause of your daytime yawns.

NARCOLEPSY

◆ *Do you feel irresistibly sleepy during the day? Do you ever have "sleep attacks" as you read, work, or drive?*

◆ *Do some or all of your muscles suddenly feel weak, particularly during times of intense emotion?*

◆ *Do you have vivid, often frightening hallucinations as you wake up or fall asleep?*

◆ *Are you sometimes unable to move when waking up or falling asleep?*

Narcolepsy is a mysterious, misunderstood, and often misdiagnosed disorder of wakefulness and sleep that affects more than 200,000 Americans. More than ten or fifteen years pass before most narcoleptics have their problem correctly identified. Researchers believe that only a third of the nation's narcoleptics have been diagnosed.

Narcolepsy is an inherited disorder that usually begins insidiously in adolescence or young adulthood; it is characterized by increasing daytime sleepiness. Regardless of how much they have slept at night, narcoleptics cannot keep their eyes open through the day. They become sleepy not just during quiet activities, like reading or watching a movie, but when speaking to others, driving their cars, and even while making love. For them, daytime sleepiness is not simply drowsiness; it is an overwhelming, irresistible weariness.

Narcolepsy has a wide range of symptoms. Some narcoleptics have both daytime sleep attacks and automatic behavior, in which they continue doing routine tasks while asleep. Some have driven in this condition, waking up on the shoulder of the road or in a neighbor's driveway. Others have continued eating or washing dishes, only to awaken when they cut themselves with knives which they have grasped by the blade rather than the handle. One woman woke up to the sound of crunching china after putting her dishes in the clothes drier.

As their symptoms progress, narcoleptics have more problems sleeping at night and awaken often, sometimes craving food and sweets. In some cases they may develop breathing problems (sleep apnea). During the transitions from wakefulness to sleep and back again, they often experience realistic and horrible sensations and visual and auditory hallucinations, such as snakes crawling over them. Sleep paralysis may occur, making it impossible for them to move or cry out.

Many narcoleptics develop another troubling daytime symptom: cataplexy, a partial or complete weakening of muscle tone. Some may become weak in the knees; others fall to the ground, unable to stay upright. Usually a certain situation or intense emotion triggers a cataplectic attack. One woman collapsed whenever she began to scold or spank her child; one stockbroker would lose all muscle tone in the excitement of negotiating a big trade.

Cataplexy may be partial or complete. Some attacks are as mild as a drooping arm or chin. Usually the narcoleptic remains conscious of words and sounds but may not remember what happened during the attack. Because intense emotion—joy or rage or frustration—triggers such attacks, many narcoleptics try to repress their feelings and avoid any display of emotion.

Many narcoleptics are confused and embarrassed by their symptoms, particularly before they know what the problem is. They are considered lazy by teachers and employers, who rail at them for sleeping at their desks or on the job. Spouses and family members may resent their frequent lapses of consciousness. In severe cases, narcoleptics are totally disabled and often isolated, unable to stay awake long enough to live any semblance of a normal life.

What causes the problem

Sleep researchers do not know the specific cause of narcolepsy, but they believe that a disorder of the sleep-wake mechanism interferes with both daytime wakefulness and nighttime sleep. The mechanism that controls REM sleep seems to be involved, and narcolepsy may occur because REM sleep bursts into normal waking periods. Sleep recordings show that narcoleptics immediately enter REM as soon as they fall asleep, whether during the day or at night. The cataplexy accompanying daytime sleep attacks may be similar to the muscle inhibition of normal REM sleep, as is the problem of sleep paralysis which occurs before and after sleep. The frightening hallucinations of narcolepsy seem to be like the images in dreams.

Some investigators suspect that the cause of narcolepsy is a biochemical defect of the central nervous system, and they have been studying the role of acetylcholine, a brain chemical involved in REM sleep. Recent studies have also found increased blood flow in the brains of narcoleptics, particularly through the brain stem, where REM sleep is regulated.

Narcolepsy is hereditary, and there is a one-in-twenty chance that the children of a narcoleptic parent will develop the problem. At Stanford University, scientists have been able to breed several generations of narcoleptic dogs. Research on these animals, who collapse into sleep when other dogs might wag their tails in joy, is providing more clues into the origins of narcolepsy.

Psychological problems seem to be a result, rather than a cause, of narcolepsy. In one sample, 29 percent of narcoleptics were found to be depressed; many expressed suicidal tendencies. The stigma attached to their symptoms makes coping more difficult; sometimes a narcoleptic is regarded as mentally retarded. The use of stimulants to stay awake may compound personality problems in narcoleptics by increasing irritability and anxiety.

What can be done

Before narcolepsy can be treated, this insidious disorder must be precisely diagnosed. Diagnosis is made on the basis of the four classic symptoms: irresistible daytime sleep attacks, cataplexy, sleep paralysis, and presleep or postsleep hallucinations. The diagnosis is confirmed by recordings at a sleep laboratory, which are essentially the same as for an all-night evaluation (see chapter 19, page 288) but are done during the day. A Multiple Sleep Latency Test (MSLT) consists of a day-long series of naps, beginning at 10:00 A.M. and every two hours thereafter. Before lying down, the person is hooked up to standard polysomnogram equipment that monitors brain waves, respiration, and heartbeat. Narcoleptics not only will fall asleep almost any time they are given an opportunity to nap in the day but will enter REM within minutes. Two episodes of daytime sleep with REM periods confirm that the problem is narcolepsy.

The sleep center also will try to rule out other causes of excessive daytime sleepiness, such as hyperthyroidism, hypoglycemia, and sleep apnea (page 192 and page 227). In a Stanford University study, 12 percent of the male narcoleptics, who also tended to be overweight and have high blood pressure, had sleep apnea as well. Researchers distinguish among different types of narcolepsy, including narcolepsy related to only REM sleep, NREM sleep, or a combination of the two.

Treatment depends on the severity of the problem. If you have mild to moderate narcolepsy, you may be able to cope with minor adjustments in your life-style. Good sleep habits, including regular bedtimes and sleeping until a spontaneous awakening, are essential. Frequent daytime naps—even as many as six ten-minute naps a day—can be extremely beneficial. Sometimes simply closing your eyes for a few minutes may prevent a sleep attack. If anyone questions your behavior, you can tell them you are meditating.

Narcoleptic sleep attacks may tend to occur cyclically, following the ninety-minute cycle of REM sleep; you might be able to time your naps accordingly. Many people tend to underestimate their own sleepiness and do not realize that they need a nap. To learn to recognize your peak times of sleepiness, keep a nap diary and record how you feel throughout the day. Some narcoleptics rely on mild stimulants like coffee to keep them awake. However, tolerance to caffeine builds up quite quickly.

In more troublesome cases, physicians prescribe a variety of medications: some are drugs with stimulating properties to overcome daytime sleepiness;

others prevent cataplectic attacks. The stimulating drugs include amphetamines, such as Desoxyn and Dexedrine. These powerful drugs may trigger serious side effects, including heart problems, headaches, psychological upsets, and personality changes, and they can be addictive. Some physicians deal with the problem of increasing tolerance and dependence by gradually withdrawing or reducing the drugs during vacations or holidays and then reinstituting therapy at a lower dose. Ritalin (methylphenidate) is a stimulant that has fewer complications. Its primary adverse reactions are nervousness and insomnia, and it can lead to drug dependence. It is widely used to treat hyperactive children, but its long-term side-effects are not known. Tests on pregnant women have not been conducted.

Other drugs, primarily antidepressants such as imipramine, are prescribed to control cataplexy. Less is known about their long-range effects than about those of stimulants. Two side effects of the antidepressants are particularly troubling for narcoleptics: sleepiness (in addition to that caused by the illness itself) and impotence. Side effects caused by high doses and complications because of interactions with other drugs may make it necessary to reduce or eliminate their use in some patients. Sudden withdrawal, however, can lead to extreme sleepiness, a dangerous degree of depression, and a dramatic increase in cataplexy. Some physicians suggest occasional withdrawal in male patients to allow a return to normal sexual activity.

Researchers are studying other medications, including Inderal (propranolol), an antihypertensive, and methysergide, a compound that reduces serotonin, the brain chemical associated with sleep. None have yet proved to be safer or more effective than current drugs.

Narcolepsy does seem to abate with age; it may be that patients learn to cope better with its symptoms and side effects over time. For help in coping, the American Narcolepsy Association (ANA), a nonprofit organization, has prepared packets of information for narcoleptics and their families, as well as a documentary film, "Keep Us Awake." This group lobbies on behalf of research and aid for narcoleptics and encourages support groups for patients and families. The ANA's address is: P.O. Box 5846, Stanford, California 94304.

BREATHING PROBLEMS
(OBSTRUCTIVE SLEEP APNEA)

• *Have you been told that you snore raucously, with momentary silences between loud, gasping snorts?*
• *Have you been told that you flail about as you sleep, often sitting up while making choking sounds?*
• *Are you so tired during the day that you black out for brief periods?*
• *Do you have headaches in the morning?*

People who stop breathing episodically during sleep because of a condition called sleep apnea are endangering life and health whenever they lay themselves down to rest. Central apnea, in which the brain stops sending signals to the diaphragm, usually leads to complaints of sleepless nights (see page 192). The victims of obstructive apnea, caused by blockage of the upper airway, become excessively sleepy during the day.

An estimated 100,000 American adults—mostly men—have obstructive apnea; male victims outnumber females by thirty to one. Apnea becomes more common with increasing age. In one study, 25 percent of otherwise healthy men over age sixty suffered from obstructive apnea.

The first clue to this breathing problem is the sound of the sleeper; people with obstructive apnea drown out most snorers. An obstruction in the airway blocks the supply of oxygen, and normal breathing stops; this is a time of ominous silence. The brain, signaled that the body needs oxygen, rouses the sleeper, usually not quite to the point of awakening so that he sucks in air loudly and vigorously. The struggle for air may be accompanied by violent movements as well as a medley of snorts, chokes, and gasps. The victim is unaware of these strange paroxysms in the night; the bed partner is the one who complains about the cacophony and commotion. In severe cases, more than 500 apneic episodes, each lasting from ten seconds to two minutes, may occur in a night. Sometimes obstructive apnea occurs along with central apnea.

Obstructive apnea devastates daytime functioning. Like narcoleptics (page 222), apnea victims are prone to sleep attacks and "microsleeps" during the day. If they fall asleep while doing routine tasks, they may continue this automatic behavior, sometimes endangering themselves and others. They may fall asleep in their seats or on their feet, often creating embarrassing situations. Like narcoleptics, they may have bizarre hallucinations as they wake up or fall asleep. Unlike narcoleptics, they never have muscle weakness (cataplexy), and daytime naps do not refresh them. Long naps, interrupted by the same breathing problems as nighttime sleep, may actually increase grogginess. Sleep attacks may become progressively worse, with victims falling asleep eating, driving, or during sexual intercourse.

Apnea can end a life; more often it erodes the quality of life. In a study of twenty-five victims, twelve reported problems of impotence, abated sexual drive, and difficulty with erection and ejaculation. The sexual problems occurred regardless of whether the patients showed any signs of depression on psychological tests. Six of the twenty-five noted personality changes, including anxiety and depression. Two blamed the breakup of their marriages on their increased hostility, irritability, and aggressiveness. Some reported puzzling episodes of jealousy and suspicion. Morning headaches occurred as often as once a week, usually disappearing in the afternoon.

Ten of the couples in the study on apnea resorted to sleeping in separate beds. The wives reported that their husbands were extremely agitated in the night, often unwittingly slapping and kicking them. Occasionally a victim would stand up, walk a few steps, and collapse. His spouse would find him asleep on the floor in the morning. Two of the men developed enuresis (see Bed-Wetting," page 204).

What causes the problem

The lack of restful sleep and a buildup of an oxygen debt (hypoxia) in the blood because of the breathing disruptions cause excessive daytime sleepiness. Some researchers believe that a dysfunction of the central nervous system is always involved in sleep apnea, whether or not the airway is blocked. Some cases of obstructive sleep apnea may be caused by extreme obesity, enlarged tonsils and adenoids, or abnormally thick tissue in the soft palate. Patients who are very heavy are sometimes referred to as having the "Pickwickian syndrome," which is named for Charles Dickens's corpulent character. Other patients have malformations of the jaw or neurological disturbances. Many apneics have very thick double chins, composed of muscle as well as fat. The most baffling cases are those in which the victims are thin and have no detectable disorders of their airways.

Obstructive apnea may be more potentially dangerous than central apnea because the breathing stoppages sometimes last longer; the sleeper seems to resist the efforts of the diaphragm to restore normal respiration. Hypoventilation (inadequate oxygen supply) may persist into the day because, as carbon dioxide builds up in the blood, it blunts the receptors that stimulate normal respiration. Chronically high carbon dioxide levels and low oxygen concentrations in the blood may lead to severe health threats, including hypertension (high blood pressure), abnormal heart rhythms, and other heart diseases. These can become life-threatening. In children, a chronic lack of oxygen may impair brain development and learning ability.

What can be done

If you have been told that you thrash about and snort in the night, place a tape recorder under your bed and listen to your nightsounds in the morning. If they sound suspicious, take the tape with you when you see a sleep specialist. Some experts can predict the diagnosis on the basis of a tape recording alone. However, most sleep centers will ask for an all-night recording (see chapter 19, page 288) to confirm the problem and to determine how severe it is. A few patients have had 800 to 900 apneic episodes recorded during a night in a sleep laboratory.

If your problem is mild and seems related to obesity, dieting may help. Sometimes corrective surgery is performed to remove large tonsils or excess fatty tissue from the soft palate. These approaches work only in a limited number of cases.

Drug therapy has not been particularly successful. Many different medications have been tried, including drugs used to relieve asthma, such as aminophylline and theophylline; however, sleep researchers disagree about their efficacy for most patients with obstructive apnea.

In serious cases in which the patients have extremely disturbed nighttime sleep and impaired daytime functioning, the recommended therapy is tracheostomy, in which surgeons create an opening in the windpipe to allow air to enter. During the day, the opening is closed to permit normal speech. This procedure can be difficult and dangerous, because victims of apnea tend to have short, thick necks that require special techniques and tubing.

The reported success with this technique has been dramatic. Excessive daytime sleepiness and morning headaches usually disappear within forty-eight hours. Some patients say they feel like themselves for the first time in years. One man said that his marriage, on the brink of a breakup, was saved. Sleep attacks, which make victims confused and suspicious, are totally eliminated. Normal sexual appetites and functioning are restored. According to long-term follow-up studies at Stanford University, all patients have returned to their jobs and have no lingering sleep problems. However, the findings on patients who *refused* the tracheostomy are grim. Most of the patients became progressively worse and eventually were disabled and bedridden. Several died in their sleep within six months of the diagnosis of obstructive sleep apnea.

MEDICAL CAUSES

* *Have you been taking pain-killing drugs or antihistamines?*
* *Do you have a chronic illness?*

Medical problems can cause sleepiness during the day as well as sleeplessness at night. Among the physical disorders that can cause sleepiness during the day are extreme obesity, hypoglycemia (commonly called low blood sugar), hypothyroidism, diabetes, nutritional deficiencies (including skipping breakfast), multiple sclerosis and other degenerative diseases, anemia, many types of infections, and injuries to the brain or nervous system. Surgery for Parkinson's disease, intractable pain, and other neurological problems can produce both excessive daytime sleepiness and abnormal sleep. The location of the surgical scars seems more significant than the initial disease in terms of effects on sleep. In both children and adults, daytime sleepiness is a common—and sometimes the only—symptom of progressive hydrocephalus, the accumulation of fluid within the skull. Sleepiness also can be a woman's first clue that she is pregnant.

Many medications can make you sleepy during the day. Cold capsules and hay fever remedies that contain antihistamines (see page 147) are common culprits. Pain-killing drugs and sedatives also may be the cause of grogginess and fatigue.

What can be done

Talk to your doctor about your sleepiness. A change in dose, timing, or brand of medication may resolve the problem. Sometimes sleepiness can be a clue to an underlying problem. If you are taking drugs that make you drowsy, be cautious when driving or operating machinery. Be especially wary of alcohol, which can dramatically enhance the effects of these drugs. And do not try to fight one drug's effects with another drug; you will only compound your problems.

DRUG-RELATED SLEEPINESS

◆ *Have you been using stimulants, including coffee and nicotine, or drugs with stimulating properties to stay alert during the day?*
◆ *Have you been taking sleeping pills or other sedatives for more than several days?*
◆ *Have you stopped taking a stimulant or sleeping pill that you used for an extended time period?*

Drugs with stimulating properties and sleeping pills can have paradoxical effects. People who take sleeping pills regularly may find themselves wide-awake at night. Stimulant users, on the other hand, may be extremely sleepy during the day. Sudden withdrawal from drugs can bring on more severe effects.

What causes the problem

USE OF AND WITHDRAWAL FROM STIMULATING DRUGS Many people rely on various "uppers" to boost their energy. Sometimes they take amphetamines and other powerful drugs; sometimes they use milder agents, like cigarettes and coffee. As any of these substances wears off, users may feel sleepy. Tolerance gradually develops, and they find themselves using larger amounts to stay alert. The longer they use stimulating drugs, the less effective they are—and the sooner their effects wear off. Throughout the day they may "crash" because of mini-withdrawals.

Sleepiness is not the only unexpected effect. Many users of stimulating drugs become irritable, lose weight, descend into deep depressions, perform automatic behaviors, and experience blackouts and amnesiac episodes. Raising the drug dosage temporarily overcomes these problems but leads to greater tolerance and increased physical dependence.

Sudden withdrawal can lead to a dramatic—but temporary—increase in daytime sleepiness. If stimulating drugs have been taken for medical reasons, the users may not understand why they suddenly feel so sleepy after their prescription runs out.

CHRONIC USE OF "DOWNERS" (Sleeping Pills, Tranquilizers, Sedatives) Drugs that dampen the body's alertness and responsiveness are colloquially called "downers." They include sleeping pills, certain anticonvulsant and antihypertension medications, antihistamines, muscle relaxants, and alcohol. These drugs may stay in the body long after they are ingested. This is particularly true in the elderly, whose metabolisms are slower.

Some people may rely on tranquilizers and sedatives to cope with stressful social or interpersonal situations. Often they do not recognize the drugs as the cause of their daytime grogginess. They also may not realize that they have become dependent on pills as props to get them through the day. Sometimes patients get "hooked" on such medications during long hospitalization or recuperation periods. Large bedtime doses of drugs that depress the central nervous system may create respiratory problems (including worsened apnea, pages 192 and 227) that enhance daytime sleepiness.

The symptoms of reliance on "downers" include grogginess, depression, irritability, shakiness, automatic behavior, agitation, amnesia, and paranoid thinking. If the drugs are taken in the evening, sleep time may be much longer than usual. Sleep recordings show less REM sleep and an increase in deep NREM sleep if the drugs are used only occasionally, but a reduction in both REM and NREM is recorded with chronic use. (Chapter 10, "The Perils of Sleeping Pills," describes how various sleeping pills affect daytime functioning.)

What can be done

It is easier to prevent than to treat these problems. Be wary of taking any drug to boost you up or bring you down. If you must take drugs that affect energy and rest for medical reasons, follow your doctor's suggestions for appropriate doses and duration of use. If you have been using uppers or downers for a long period of time, seek professional help in breaking the habit (see chapter 10, page 149). Do not try to quit "cold turkey." Withdrawal may lead to frightening extremes of daytime sleepiness and nighttime sleeplessness. You should wean yourself gradually from these drugs, under the close supervision of a physician.

PERIODIC HYPERSOMNIA (KLEINE-LEVIN SYNDROME)

- *Do you go through periods of excessive sleep with intermittent times of normal sleep?*
- *Do you experience periodic binges of excessive eating, sexual activity, and sleep?*

Sometimes excessive daytime sleepiness waxes and wanes over several weeks or months. If you feel that you go through cycles of extreme tiredness, keep a sleep diary for several weeks so you can identify the times of greatest sleepiness.

The Kleine-Levin Syndrome is an extremely rare disorder that occurs most often in male adolescents. Its victims go through recurrent periods of excessive sleep, withdrawing from social contacts and retiring to bed whenever possible. Sometimes they become irritable, confused, voraciously hungry, and sexually uninhibited.

What causes the problem

This seems to be a disorder of the appetite-control centers in the brain. Sometimes victims eat nothing or devour huge amounts of food. Or they may speak incoherently, become delusional, or sexually exhibit themselves. Unexplained fevers may occur, and there may be metabolic disturbances that can be detected by urine analysis. Physical or emotional stress or fevers may precipitate a period of excessive sleep. While most of the victims are male, Kleine-Levin syndrome may be diagnosed in females.

Generally this syndrome is ascribed to an intermittent defect or dysfunction in the brain. The precise cause of the bizarre symptoms is unknown. During the intervening periods of alertness, there uually are no signs of physical or psychiatric disturbance. There tend to be several attacks, each lasting for several weeks, during the year. The syndrome is generally first experienced between ages ten and twenty-one; the victims usually outgrow this disorder by age forty with no residual complications.

Researchers suspect some periodic hyperreactivity in certain regions of the brain related to sex hormones. Except during the binge periods, the young men with this problem tend to be abnormally shy and withdrawn. Sleep recordings show that victims have less REM and less deep NREM sleep. REM periods may occur quite early in the night, in a pattern similar to that of depressed persons.

What can be done

Little is known about how to prevent or control this baffling problem. Some physicians have reported that lithium carbonate, a drug often used in treating manic-depressive illness (which is characterized by cyclic mood shifts), may prevent but not end the attacks.

OTHER HYPERSOMNIAS

◆ *Do you experience "microsleeps," brief periods of lapsed consciousness, during the day?*
◆ *Do you have problems completing complex tasks during the day?*
◆ *Do you have problems complying with any fixed schedule?*
◆ *Do you feel pessimistic about your future and uninterested in your health, appearance, or friends?*

SUBWAKEFULNESS People with this problem have normal amounts of undisturbed nocturnal sleep, with normal REM and NREM periods, but still are sleepy throughout the day. They frequently report lapses in consciousness that last less than a minute (called "microsleeps") apparent failures of memory, and difficulty in concentration.

This rare disorder may be caused by abnormal arousal mechanisms in the brain. When tested, the spinal fluid of victims contains unusually low concentrations of a substance identified as homovanillic acid (HVA), a product of the brain chemical dopamine. This may indicate that they lack sufficient amounts of dopamine to keep them alert.

NEUTRAL STATE SYNDROME In this problem, both the sleep-inducing and wakefulness mechanisms seem disordered. Like people with subwakefulness, victims are extremely drowsy and fall into frequent microsleeps during the day. While they can perform simple, repetitive tasks, they cannot complete more complex duties. Because of the frequent blackouts during the day, they experience amnesia and are unable to recall their activities. Unlike those with subwakefulness, they have aroused nocturnal sleep with hundreds of "micro-wakes" lasting ten to sixty seconds. They seem doubly cursed: unable to work by day and incapable of sleeping through the night.

HYPERSOMNIA *with abnormal central nervous system findings* These persons, sleepy throughout the day, have a distinct abnormality that can be detected by laboratory tests of their spinal fluid: they have unusually high levels of a substance identified as 5-hydroxyindoleactectic acid (5-HIAA). This is a metabolic end-product of serotonin, a neurotransmitter or messenger chemical in the brain that is associated with sleep. The high levels of this substance may indicate much higher than normal amounts of serotonin. This problem is treated with drugs that inhibit serotonin production.

ABNORMAL SLEEP-WAKE RHYTHMS A biological clock out of synch with the rest of the world can create problems of daytime sleepiness as well as nighttime sleeplessness. People out of phase with the normal twenty-four-hour rhythm can sleep normally—but not at times others consider normal. Their problem may be delayed sleep onset (page 179) or a sleep-wake cycle that is longer than twenty-four hours or highly irregular (page 180).

PSYCHOLOGICAL FACTORS People of all ages may become extremely sleepy during the day and tend to feel a need for daytime naps because of psychological problems. Excessive sleepiness is reported in the initial stages of depression in which the patient's moods shift from manic highs to disturbing lows. People with this sort of depression may sleep a normal amount of time or awaken early in the morning (page 214), yet they never feel refreshed by sleep. Depressed children and adolescents are likely to sleep more rather than less, and usually there are other changes in appetite and behavior. A careful psychiatric examination is needed to diagnose and treat the underlying problem.

MIXED HYPERSOMNIA This disorder combines features of other hypersomnias: excessive daytime sleepiness, cataplexy (muscle weakness), and occasional REM periods during daytime sleep. Unlike narcoleptics, its victims have an adequate amount of undisturbed nocturnal sleep and seem to have daytime disturbances of both REM and NREM sleep. Usually victims are given stimulating drugs to keep them alert during the day.

IDIOPATHIC HYPERSOMNIA Individuals with this problem may stay in bed as long as twenty hours a night yet still suffer strong but *resistible* daytime sleepiness. In making a diagnosis, physicians first rule out brain tumors, head injuries, strokes, emotional problems, and sleep-wake rhythm disorders. In one study of such patients, 33 percent had sleep drunkenness (page 217) for fifteen to sixty minutes after waking. Their heart rates were higher than normal before and during sleep, and their sleep seemed more aroused. Even when they sleep for twenty hours, they progress normally through ninety-minute NREM-REM cycles. Some doctors prescribe daytime stimulating drugs for these patients.

SUBJECTIVE HYPERSOMNIA *without objective findings* Patients with subjective hypersomnia complain about daytime sleepiness, but clinical evaluation and sleep latency tests show no abnormalities. Often patients report impaired functioning for one to five years, but physical and psychological assessments are normal. The problem may start when a job or other responsibilities require regular hours of wakefulness and sleep. Researchers describe these patients as "passive, perplexed individuals" seeking confirmation of their problem as well as treatment for it. It may be that current tests are not sensitive or sophisticated enough to measure and evaluate their sleepiness, or they may be confusing their sleepiness with other physical sensations. They may have unusual sensitivity to irregular sleep and waking habits or a hidden disorder of their sleep-wake cycle. Or they may be so overly concerned about their sleep that they conclude there must be a problem even when there is none.

INADEQUATE SLEEP This cause seems so obvious it hardly merits a mention. However, many people underestimate their true sleep needs, limit their time in bed, and then wonder why they are struggling to stay awake during the day. Some sleep researchers suggest that millions of us may be guilty of deliberate sleep-deprivation. In our relentless, fast-paced, round-the-clock society, we trim hours off our sleep time to allow time for other pursuits. All too often we end up shortchanging our energy and our health. Some people may brag that they can "get by" on five or six hours of sleep; others turn to stimulants to help them make it through the day. However, most people find it difficult to maintain this sort of schedule for long.

CHAPTER 16

Bad Nights: Occasional Sleep Problems

◆ *If you are sleeping in an unfamiliar setting or are going through a time of intense stress, see "Situational Problems," page 238.*

◆ *If you have been flying across several time zones, see "Jet Lag," page 239.*

◆ *If you work nights or evenings or rotate shifts, see "Shift Work," page 241:*

◆ *If you awaken because of physical discomfort, have a chronic illness, or are taking medications for a medical problem, see "Illness and Injury," page 243.*

◆ *If you are sleepier during the day or sleep less at night than before you became pregnant, see "Pregnancy/Postpartum," page 249.*

◆　　◆　　◆

"I t's been one of those days." How often have you said this to explain a day in which nothing went right? Just as you will experience days of baffling difficulty, you will also have some nights during which you cannot sleep as you usually do.

Often the circumstances are beyond your control: travel, jet lag, work shifts, medical problems, life crises. However, if you do not understand what is happening to your sleep and why, you may overreact to your sleeplessness—and end up with a chronic sleep problem. This chapter cannot guarantee that you will have no more bad nights, but it should help you make it through "one of those nights."

SITUATIONAL PROBLEMS

- *Are you sleeping in an unfamiliar setting?*
- *Are you going through a time of intense stress?*
- *Has your problem developed in the last three weeks?*

Everybody has an occasional bad night, and the most common cause is a strange sleep environment. Whether you are traveling for business or pleasure, it may be difficult for you to sleep well in a hotel, motel, or friend's home. If you have crossed several time zones en route to your night's lodging, you are likely to have even more problems (see page 239). Some travelers rely on familiar rituals that they use at home or on trips; others take a few familiar objects with them. A portable alarm clock may be the answer to concern about the front desk forgetting to call you on time; a small radio may help lull you to sleep. Be sure to take some relaxing reading materials in case you have problems falling asleep. If all else fails, console yourself by remembering that a night of poor sleep is *not* a serious threat to your daytime performance or well-being. Don't let yourself nap the next day, and you should be so sleepy at bedtime that you will drift into sleep as if you were back in your own bed.

Sometimes a situation rather than a location keeps you awake at night. Millions of children have problems falling asleep every December 24; adults are more likely to have sleep problems the night before a wedding or big exam or job interview. In these instances, the problem is an overactive arousal system. Soothing sleep rituals may help you relax and fall asleep; the relaxation therapies described in Chapter 9 can help you cope with overarousal before sleep and during the night.

Because sleep mirrors your daytime emotions, any trauma—death of a loved one, a family illness, divorce, a painful life transition—is likely to disrupt sleep. The greater the emotional impact, the more disturbed your sleep may be. During a family crisis, many individuals are affected around the clock. Even when they go for long periods without sleep, they are too agitated during the day to nap. They feel exhausted, edgy, and achy. This grueling sleeplessness can greatly affect physical and psychological health. Most physicians feel that a time of great difficulty for an individual is one of the few times when sleeping pills should be prescribed for several nights.

JET LAG

- *Have you crossed more than one time zone in your day's journey?*
- *Are you finding it hard to fall asleep or wake up at the appropriate times in your new location?*
- *Are you having difficulty accomplishing even simple tasks?*

Jet lag is a truly man-made malady. Space Age planes can zip across continents and oceans in a matter of hours; our Stone Age bodies have to struggle to catch up. "Jet lag" describes this period of adjustment when body and mind are temporarily off-cue. For occasional travelers, it is a temporary malaise; for plane crews, it is an occupational hazard.

When you travel through time zones, you can reset your watch in a matter of minutes. However, your body needs a full day per time zone to readjust, because the body's internal clockworks determine the timing of dozens of physiological processes (see chapter 2, "Sunrise, Sunset," page 24). If you arrive in London on a flight from Chicago, the time according to Big Ben may be 9:00 A.M. but according to your body clock, it is 4:00 A.M.

Jet lag is more than weariness; it is a period of subpar mental and physical functioning. Traveling east to west creates fewer problems, probably because it is easier to extend your day and stay up longer than to try to fall asleep earlier, as you must when traveling eastward. Research shows that sleep stages are dramatically different on the first night after a long transcontinental or transoceanic flight and that REM sleep is delayed and shortened. A more normal sleep pattern reappears on the second night, but sleep still tends to be fragmented and brief. You are likely to wake up at dawn unable to return to sleep, and it may take five days to adjust your sleep pattern. The older you are, the more difficult it will be. Body temperature rhythms may not become synchronized with the new schedule for a week.

Even on the fastest new planes, jet lag cannot be avoided. However, some of its effects can be minimized. Among the commonsense guidelines suggested by sleep specialists are:

- *Begin the time shift before you leave home.* You will have more problems adjusting if you have been following a rigid schedule of eating and sleeping up until the day of the flight. A week before you leave for Europe or the South Pacific, set one clock in your house to the time zone of your destination. Gradually begin going to bed and getting up earlier if you will be traveling east or staying up later if you are heading west.

• *Leave home rested.* Try to avoid last-minute haste, especially frantic packing the night before your departure and a mad rush to the airport.

• *Dress comfortably* for the plane trip. Take off your shoes during the flight. Do not try to do last-minute work on the plane.

• *Stretch occasionally.* Get up and walk. Alternately tense and relax your muscles.

• *Travel with a friend* if possible; companionship eases the tedium of a long flight.

• *Eat lightly* during the flight and for a few days afterward.

• *Do not drink, or drink lightly.* If you wish to drink, limit yourself to a glass of wine or a beer, or you may add a hangover to your jet lag problems.

• *Do not smoke, or smoke infrequently.* Cigarettes irritate eyes, ears, and throat in the zero-humidity of a plane.

• *Drink water and fruit juice*, rather than coffee, tea, and cola drinks.

• *Schedule your arrival late in the day*, close to the time of your bedtime at home. Whenever you arrive, spend a quiet first day.

• On a short trip, *stay on your home time.* Eat and sleep at the hours you normally do.

• On longer trips, *start living by the new time frame immediately.* When in Rome, sleep when the Romans do. When in New Guinea, set your watch by the local clocks.

• If you are traveling halfway around the world, *stop for a one or two-day rest.*

• *Rely on sleep rituals* (page 101) and relaxation exercises (page 113) to ease you into sleep. Avoid alcohol and sleeping pills because they may have a greater and longer effect on your sleep than the trip itself. Sleeping pills will not counter jet lag; they will only mask it.

A more complex approach to jet lag involves the use of certain types of food to influence your body's sense of time. Developed by Charles Ehret of Argonne National Laboratory in Illinois, this plan has been tested and proved effective in tests with American soldiers flown from the United States to Europe for NATO maneuvers. The anti-jet-lag strategy for a west-to-east flight begins four days prior to departure, when you "feast," eating a large, high-protein breakfast and lunch and a large dinner rich in carbohydrates. The next day you "fast," eating three skimpy, low-calorie, low-carbohydrate meals, just enough food to ward off feelings of dizziness or weakness. The next day is another time for feasting on large meals. The day of your flight you fast again, eating little and avoiding coffee and carbohydrates. The moment you board your plane, you set your watch to the local time at your destination. You avoid eating a heavy meal on the plane, and you try to rest; it may be difficult to sleep because of the nonstop chatter of other passengers and the activity of the airline crew. If you are arriving in Europe early in the morning—the most typical schedule for American travelers—try to eat a high-protein breakfast and drink coffee before landing (you can ask the stewardess to save the dinner you refused earlier for this meal). After you disembark, take your time collecting your luggage, going through customs, and reaching your hotel. At noon eat a large lunch, high in protein. For dinner, eat an ample meal that is high in carbohydrates rather than protein. Go to bed at the appropriate local time and get up at a normal time, even if you have not slept well. This scheme does not eliminate jet lag, but it does minimize its aftereffects. For your own sake, plan a quiet, relaxed schedule for the first two or three days of your trip.

SHIFT WORK

+ *Do you work nights or evenings?*
+ *Do you rotate shifts?*
+ *Do you readjust your schdule on weekends and during vacations?*

More than 13.5 million Americans—18 percent of the work force—are part-time or full-time evening and night workers. Their jobs are as diversified as the jobs of their daytime counterparts: engineers, pilots, factory workers, doctors, truck drivers, entertainers, computer programmers, communications specialists, air traffic controllers, cooks, cleaners, nurses, sailors, and dozens more. Whatever their job, night workers tend to have a common problem: sleep.

Research has shown that shift workers get less sleep than others. They average only 5.6 hours of sleep every 24 hours, compared to 7.5 hours for the general population. Rarely do they sleep more than 7 hours at a stretch; often they wake up after 4 or 5 hours, unrefreshed but unable to go back to sleep. The result is chronic fatigue, psychological troubles, and increased vulnerability to disease.

These problems are caused by disruptions in your circadian (daily) rhythms. Whether you punch in at dawn or at dusk, your internal clock will follow its set rhythm, and your body temperature, blood pressure, and other physiological functions will rise and fall at their accustomed pace. It takes several weeks for your body to adjust to a 180° shift in schedule.

Sometimes this adjustment is never made, even after months or years on the evening or night shift. One reason is that workers find it all but impossible to sleep during the day because of light, noise, ringing telephones, or crying children. On weekends they may shift back to a normal daytime routine so they can spend time with their families and friends. The result of these fluctuations is chronic dissynchronization. With no constant rhythm to their sleep-wake cycles, shift workers may live continually off balance.

The problem is greater for people who rotate shifts often. These workers are more likely to have accidents on the job, to report marital and sexual problems, and to develop health problems. They seem particularly prone to digestive ailments, perhaps because their schedule is not well timed to the rhythmic release of digestive enzymes and acids. Shift workers also drink more alcohol (often to fall asleep), take more sleeping pills, and use more tobacco and caffeine (often to stay awake). Some of the subsequent ill-effects, particularly sleep difficulties, may persist long after their schedules become fixed.

Some experts are suggesting new guidelines for scheduling shift rotations. For routine jobs, daily shifts may be better than weekly ones. Workers would report for the day shift on Monday, switch to evenings on Tuesday, work nights on Wednesday, and take Thursday off. Friday, they again work during the day. This schedule, popular in Europe, allows employees to stay tuned to a standard time frame and to eat at least one meal a day with their families. For jobs that require more concentration or decision-making abilities, much longer shifts, of months rather than days or weeks, may be better because they allow the body clock to catch up with the time clock.

The ability of individuals to adjust to erratic or unusual schedules varies greatly. Young people seem far more resilient than older individuals; people over the age of fifty generally should try to avoid irregular hours. Employees with digestive problems or with medical conditions (like diabetes) that require regular food intake or medications also should avoid shift work.

The following are practical steps you can take if you are working nights or rotating shifts:

• Try to *eat your meals at the same time* every day in order to make as little change in your circadian rhythms as possible.

• Try to *sleep at least four hours during the same time each day.* If you are working nights and usually go to sleep at 8:00 A.M., do the same on Saturday and Sunday but get up at noon if you want to see your family and friends.

• When you try to sleep during the day, *darken the room* with heavy draperies.

• Experiment with ways to *block out daytime noise.* Ear plugs, "white noise" machines (page 79), or the hum of an air conditioner or fan may help. You might also consider soundproofing the bedroom.

• *Restrict your use of stimulants.* Do not drink coffee, tea, or cola drinks or smoke heavily in the hours before going to bed. Eliminate other forms of stimulation, such as watching an exciting sports event or vigorous exercise, before your bedtime.

• *Do not try to shift gears* by changing your wake-sleep schedule on weekends or brief holidays. Your body will be more confused by the erratic timing than it was when you shifted to evening or night work.

• Try to *relieve the strain* of your unusual work schedule on your family. Your spouse and children may resent your absence at night and your demands for quiet during the day. Talk about these issues; enlist your family's help in finding ways and times to spend a few hours a day together.

ILLNESS AND INJURY

• *Do you awaken because of pain, itching, or other discomforts?*
• *Are you recovering from an injury, illness, or operation?*
• *Do you have a chronic illness?*
• *Are you taking medications for your medical problem?*

The diseases that plague us during the day do not rest at night. They relentlessly disrupt our sleep just when we may feel we need it most. Sometimes disturbed sleep is the earliest clue to a physical problem; sometimes it is a lingering symptom. The relationship between illness and sleep varies. In some instances, a sleep problem is the direct consequence of a medical or surgical condition or treatment. Some medical disorders worsen in sleep; others improve. Whenever a disease or injury is the cause of a sleep disturbance, the only hope for a good night's sleep is treating the underlying problem.

The most common cause of sleep disturbance is pain. People with arthritis or rheumatism are most likely to awaken in the night, probably because of the discomfort caused by their body movements. Another common symptom, itching, can keep you awake all night long. Researchers cannot confirm that pain and itching actually get worse during the night; you simply may notice them more because there is nothing that distracts you. If these symptoms are keeping you awake at night, see your physician. Long-acting medications may be the key to sleeping through the nights until you recover.

Almost any illness, from a common cold to a life-threatening malady, may disrupt sleep. The following discussions cover the most common sleep-disturbing disorders, grouped according to the organs and systems they affect.

Central Nervous System

Sleep may be disrupted because of disturbances in the brain; brain tumors; vascular problems, such as migraine headaches; infections, such as encephalitis; degenerative conditions, such as Parkinson's disease or multiple sclerosis; and injury to the brain. Epilepsy and headache are the two most common conditions that disturb sleep.

EPILEPSY Nighttime epileptic seizures are common in people with this brain disorder. In some patients, seizures occur almost exclusively at night. Attacks of such "sleep epilepsy" usually happen in the first two hours after bedtime or between 4:00 A.M. and 6:00 A.M. Convulsive seizures usually cause bladder and bowel incontinence.

Sleep-related epileptic seizures may occur at any age but are most frequent in children. Occasionally a child may have 30 to 100 small seizures a night, but parents often mistake them for body movements. Sleep seizures occur in 20 to 25 percent of patients who also have seizures during the day. About 10 percent of patients have a family history of epilepsy, but familial "sleep epilepsy" is rare.

Any occurrence of sleep seizures should be evaluated by a physician. Epilepsy is a complex and varied disease, and it is difficult to generalize about the course of implications of sleep-related seizures. Usually they lead to no daytime impairments, but they may give rise to behaviors that mimic such sleep disorders as sleepwalking, bed-wetting, leg jerks, and breathing difficulties. If the sleep seizures are related to organic brain disease, the patient may have neurological or intelligence deficits as well as psychological problems.

VASCULAR HEADACHES Tension headaches are daytime phenomena; headaches involving the blood vessels disturb sleep. Sleep-related cluster headaches are severe, unilateral (affecting only one side) headaches that appear in an on-off pattern of attacks during sleep. They usually awaken the sleeper during the night or early in the morning, and they occur during sleep, even when the sleep schedule is shifted. Another type of sleep-related headache is chronic paroxysmal hemicrania, a unilateral headache characterized by more frequent but briefer attacks.

Both types of headache may appear during the day but seem to become worse at night, particularly during REM sleep. Paroxysmal hemicrania appears only during REM periods, disturbing sleep in the early morning. The association with REM suggests that physiological changes triggered by REM, particularly in blood pressure, may be responsible. Because the arteries in the head are distended and squeezed, the pain can be agonizing.

Researchers do not know why these headaches occur only in some individuals. There does seem to be a familial predisposition, but neither type of headache appears before puberty. Women are slightly more likely to suffer these headaches and tend to have more severe pain. Cluster headaches may endure for hours; hemicranias last only five to fifteen minutes but may occur more than twenty times in a day. Unpublished reports suggest that REM-suppressing drugs taken before sleep can reduce the number of attacks.

Respiratory system

Sleep apnea is the most serious respiratory problem related to sleep (see pages 192 and 227). However, any chronic obstructive lung disease, such as emphysema, affects and is affected by sleep. The decrease in oxygen levels during sleep may exacerbate these disorders.

ASTHMA This chronic respiratory disease, characterized by attacks of breathlessness, wheezing, and coughing up of sputum, often becomes worse in the night. Nocturnal asthma attacks usually occur after several hours of sleep, particularly after the deep NREM sleep of the early night. Researchers do not know why asthma flares up in the night, but the incidence of asthmatic attacks actually seems higher in the evening and night than during the day. The reason could be the circadian rhythm for the release of substances involved in an asthma attack. Lying flat also may increase airway resistance and interfere with breathing. Perhaps dreaming or the physiological changes associated with REM periods trigger some attacks.

Heart and blood vessels

More deaths from cardiac disorders occur during the night than during the day. Half of all heart attacks happen at night; strokes occur more often during sleep than during wakefulness. Physicians have long realized that these facts must represent more than mere coincidence and have puzzled over what happens to the heart when the sleeper lies down to rest.

Heart rate and blood pressure normally change dramatically in different sleep stages; these changes can be hazardous in patients with vulnerable or impaired hearts. Some people develop dyspnea, or shortage of breath; this may be caused simply by the act of lying down rather than by sleep itself. Other problems include angina, hypertension, arrhythmias, and congestive heart failure.

ANGINA (*Chest Pain*) For decades medical scientists have speculated about the connection between dreams and angina attacks. An emotionally charged dream might well trigger the sort of physiological responses that lead to angina, but studies have not confirmed this direct relationship. Most physicians prescribe standard angina pain-relieving medications at bedtime to deal with this symptom.

HYPERTENSION (*High Blood Pressure*) Normal blood pressure in adults is 120 systolic pressure (the pressure when the heart contracts) and 80 diastolic pressure (between contractions). Hypertension, one of the leading risk factors of heart disease, occurs when the artery walls squeeze down excessively on the blood flowing by. Blood pressure is elevated during REM periods of sleep, perhaps increasing the risk to hypertensive patients. Some sleep researchers believe that sleep apnea, in which breathing stops and oxygen levels drop intermittently in the night, may help cause or exacerbate hypertension.

CARDIAC ARRHYTHMIAS *(Irregular Heartbeats)* For reasons researchers do not yet understand, the heart may beat erratically—and even stop beating—during sleep. Simultaneous sleep apnea and cardiopulmonary stress may be the cause of some arrhythmias. Stanford University researchers also have discovered that the heart can stop contracting (a condition called asystole) in otherwise healthy adults.

CONGESTIVE HEART FAILURE/PULMONARY EDEMA When the heart's pumping capacity is well below normal, fluid begins to collect in the lungs and extremities. The heart is then said to be "in failure." If this happens during the night, the person may sit up with a feeling of suffocation, gasping for air. These episodes may be avoided or minimized by sleeping in a sitting position.

If this problem becomes severe, a medical emergency—pulmonary edema—may develop, and the patient will cough and wheeze. This is a serious, life-threatening crisis, and you should get medical help if your difficulty in breathing and feeling of congestion become worse.

Digestive system

ULCERS You may well have awakened in the night with indigestion after an exotic meal or a spicy pizza. However, most of the time, secretion of gastric acid decreases during sleep—except in ulcer patients. Some studies have shown that ulcer patients secrete three to twenty times more gastric acid in their sleep than normal subjects. Some physicians advise their ulcer patients to take antacids before bed; others suggest a glass of milk. The advent of a very effective drug for treating ulcers—Tagamet (cimetidine)—has greatly decreased sleep problems for people with severe ulcer disease.

GASTROESOPHAGEAL REFLUX People with this disorder wake up with a burning pain in their throats and a sour taste in their mouths. They also may cough, choke, and feel vague respiratory discomforts. Often these people have no daytime symptoms; the reason for their nocturnal symptoms is regurgitation of stomach acid into the esophagus.

The cause of this disorder may be unusually low pressure at the sphincter, or end, of the lower esophagus. Both men and women can be affected, and there seems to be no genetic pattern. Symptoms become more severe over time and can lead to serious complications, including aspiration pneumonia and increased asthma. Try eating dinner earlier, so food is digested before bedtime. Or you might try stomach-soothing over-the-counter medications to see if they help. If the problem persists, see your physician.

Reproductive system

MENSTRUATION Generally adult women do not have sleep changes related to their menstrual cycles. However, some women spend more time in REM sleep late in the cycle when they are most likely to have other premenstrual changes and symptoms. Adolescent girls may become excessively sleepy at the end of their menstrual cycles, perhaps because of increased levels of the hormone progesterone.

PAINFUL ERECTIONS On occasion, nighttime erections may be accompanied by pain so intense that it awakens the sleeper. Since erections regularly occur during REM sleep, this may be a disorder of REM-controlling mechanisms. Victims have little or no difficulty with sexual functioning when awake, and their daytime erections are not painful. Occasionally a painful erection during sleep is a sign of an anatomical defect or disease of the penis. Anxiety is usually the result, not the cause, of the problem.

Other diseases and treatments

Among the other medical conditions that can cause sleep problems are: kidney failure; diabetes; thyroid conditions; infections (bacterial, fungal, viral, and parasitic); allergies to foods, chemicals, or dust; anemia; and nutritional deficiencies.

Sometimes medical treatments cause more problems than the actual illness. Traction, casts, splints, and bulky bandages can be so uncomfortable that they interfere with sleep. If you are forced to stay in one position, you may fidget because your normal sleep movements are restricted. The anxiety of hospitalization, along with frequent awakenings as staff personnel check on intravenous lines or administer medications, can keep you awake day and night. Patients in intensive care or cardiac care units often suffer severe sleep deprivation because of the constant activity involved in their treatment. Some doctors have speculated that a patient's lack of deep, continuous sleep may impair the healing process.

Different prescription drugs affect the sleep-wake cycle in different ways. Some prolong the time needed to fall asleep. Some fragment sleep by causing multiple arousals in the night. Some lead to early morning awakenings and excessive daytime sleepiness. Among the medications implicated as sleep-disrupters are: nasal decongestants, oral contraceptives, antihypertension agents, antiasthmatics, steriods, anti–arrhythmia drugs for heart patients, cancer chemotherapy drugs, thyroid drugs, anticonvulsant drugs for epileptics, methysergide (a headache remedy), some antidepressants, and amphetamines and similar compounds.

If you suspect that a therapy or drug is interfering with your sleep, inform your doctor. A lower dose, a different time of administration, or a different medication may help you rest more easily without compromising your health. However, sometimes your physician may face a dilemma in balancing your sleep needs with proper treatment for your medical problem. There may not be an easy solution, but a carefully planned drug regimen should minimize sleep disturbances.

PREGNANCY/POSTPARTUM

- *Have you become much sleepier during the day since you became pregnant?*
- *Do you wake up often because you are too hot or too cold?*
- *Do you wake up often to urinate?*
- *Are you disturbed by dreams of having a deformed baby?*

Sleeping for two tends to be more complicated than solitary slumber. Early in pregnancy, you are likely to feel sleepy late in the afternoon and need a nap. Most mothers-to-be add an hour or more to their daily sleep time. Heed your body's signals of its need for more rest, and do not shortchange yourself or your baby of the sleep you both need.

Sleep may become more problematic as you approach delivery. By the last trimester, it may be difficult for you to find a comfortable position in bed. Your large abdomen may make sleeping on your back or face-down difficult, while lying on one side may drag you over into another awkward position. One suggestion is to try to prop yourself up, using two or three extra pillows, or to lie on your side with a pillow under your abdomen.

Pregnant women may develop "restless legs" (page 176) and have problems in falling asleep. The movements of the fetus may make it difficult to stay asleep. Some mothers insist that their babies are "night owls" and move around more at night than during the day. However, you may notice the activity more simply because of the lack of distractions. As the growing fetus presses on your bladder, you will need to urinate more during the day and night. If trips to the bathroom are disrupting your sleep, try to abstain from liquids for three or four hours before bedtime.

Pregnancy also changes your metabolic rate, often creating problems for your body's temperature control system. You may feel alternately too hot and too cold through the night. Try not to throw off all the covers at once when you wake up sweating in the night. Wait a few minutes to see if the feeling subsides. If it does not subside, gradually reduce the number of blankets. Work out an arrangement that is comfortable for your husband as well as for you. This may be as simple as his wearing thermal underwear or a robe as well as pajamas so you can eliminate a blanket or comforter.

Many pregnant women have upsetting dreams about labor and delivery. Rarely do they dream of having a normal, healthy baby who looks and acts like a baby; they are much more likely to dream of an enormous or deformed baby or even of giving birth to a litter of animals. Such dreams are normal and perhaps helpful in releasing your anxieties about the upcoming birth. One research group found that women who had anxious dreams about delivery actually had shorter labor times that those who denied their fears by "forgetting" such bad dreams.

Since any drug you take during pregnancy may affect the fetus as well, you should be wary of all sleep-inducing medications, prescription or nonprescription. Consult your obstetrician if you have been using sleeping pills or tranquilizers. If you are tempted to take a pill because you are worried about not getting enough sleep, simply try resting instead. Lying quietly for an extra hour or two will do just as much for your baby as extra sleep—without the potential dangers of pills. If you are taking medication because of a chronic sleep disorder, be sure to inform your doctor about it. A narcoleptic woman, for example, may decide not to use stimulants during pregnancy because of the potential risks to her baby. Recent research has also revealed that the use of alcohol and caffeine endangers the fetus during pregnancy.

Sleep problems do not disappear when your baby is born. In many instances, a new mother may be weary, not radiant. Delivery is a physiological upheaval, and it may take several weeks for your body and its hormones to return to normal. In the meantime, these internal changes, along with the demands of an infant for regular feedings, will disrupt your normal sleep-wake cycle. Some physicians have theorized that sleep loss may play a role in postpartum depression, and they urge new mothers to rest as much as they can.

CHAPTER 17

Children's Sleep Problems:
The Sleep of the Innocent

◆ *If your child seems exceptionally sleepy during the day and still wets the bed after age five, see "Narcolepsy," page 271.*

◆　◆　◆

No sound is more plaintive—or perplexing—to parents than their child's cry in the night. Is the baby hungry or in pain? Is the toddler having a terrible dream? Has the four-year-old wet the bed? Could the eight-year-old have fallen down the stairs while sleepwalking?

At night all of us become more vulnerable, more childlike in our fears and needs. Our children, faces damp with midnight tears, seem both more needy and more demanding than they do by day. Many parents find it difficult to understand and cope with their children's night cries and sleep problems. Yet the way you respond to a child's disturbed sleep may have lifelong effects, because you help shape your child's attitude toward sleep.

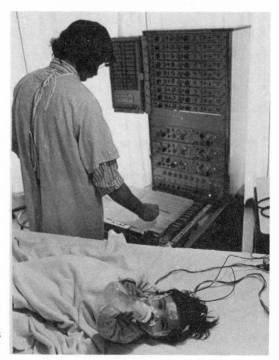

This 6-month-old child is being examined for breathing disorders during sleep at the Stanford University Sleep Research Center (California). Courtesy Stanford University News and Publications Service.

Making It Through the Night

How children sleep

As grown-ups, if our sleep has been particularly deep and refreshing, we say we slept like babies. Actually, babies sleep much differently than adults or older children. A premature baby may spend 70 percent of sleep-time in active REM-like sleep; a newborn's REM periods occupy half of its sleep. Are infants dreaming through these times? Probably not as we do. Researchers suggest that the REM periods of the very young—beginning when the fetus is still in the womb—may provide essential stimulation for the brain to develop. By generating activity in the nervous system, REM sleep may make up for the baby's relatively unstimulating environment and may play a critical role in learning processes. Infants with congenital brain impairments tend to spend less time in REM sleep than healthy newborns.

A baby's normal cycle of REM and NREM sleep—forty-five to fifty minutes—is about half as long as an adult's. A newborn seems incapable of consolidating sleep into long periods lasting several hours; instead it "naps" around the clock. From birth, individuals have enormously varied sleep needs. Some infants sleep twenty hours a day; others spend less than ten hours asleep. Throughout childhood, boys and girls mature differently by night as well as by day. These differences show up in sleep patterns as well as in daytime behavior.

From birth until age six, the brain triples in size. The intense activity of the central nervous system during this period affects the way a child perceives sleep. Children do not drift smoothly into slumber the way adults do. Because their brain cells "let go" of control unevenly, the child may feel a sudden jerk at sleep-onset that creates a very real and scary sense of falling. If we experienced this sensation, we'd probably wake up; a child usually continues to sleep but remembers the unpleasant feeling.

Children spend much more time in the deepest stages of sleep—NREM Stages 3 and 4—than adults. These periods, occurring early in the night, are when growth hormone reaches peak levels in the blood; these sleep stages are crucial for normal development. Abused children who are too frightened to sleep through the night may stop growing; this failure to thrive may be linked to the loss of deep sleep. Some of the most common disorders of children's sleep are related to the amount of time spent in this profound state of unconsciousness.

Misunderstanding of children's sleep problems can lead to nightly bedtime battles. Parents, nerves frayed because of a trying day, order a child to bed; the child refuses; the lines are drawn; the war of wills begins. There are no winners in these conflicts. Both parents and child end up exhausted and exasperated. Sometimes parents underestimate their children's fear of sleep. From the ages of two to five, boys and girls may not be able to distinguish dreams from reality. The darkness of the bedroom may scare them; they feel pangs of separation from mother. And they may recall the vivid dream image of a tiger or monster, who perhaps is still lurking between the sheets or under the bed.

These fears, along with normal tiredness, make children regress. A four-year-old will wail like a two-year-old; even school-age children may seem particularly babyish at bedtime. Parents who overreact to these normal displays of feelings that their children do not know how to articulate may reinforce unwanted behavior. Children who figure out that they can get more attention at bedtime or during the night than they do during the day will continue whatever it was that brought their parents running to their beds.

Understanding the causes of your children's sleep problems will help you cope better—and sleep better yourself. Certain disorders appear at specific stages of development. The following is a general preview of what to expect:

♦ *Infancy:*
Problems of colic, persistent night feeding, persistent night crying
♦ *Age One to Three:*
Difficulty falling asleep and waking up
"Fighting" sleep because of fears of separation or losing bladder control
Autoerotic activity, including thumb-sucking, rocking, and masturbation
    (these are normal behaviors)
Frightening dreams
♦ *Age Four to Six:*
Fears about separation and loss of control
Fear of death
Bed-wetting
Sleepwalking
Night terrors
Rocking, head-banging

Making It Through the Night

◆ *Age Six to Twelve:*
"Can't sleep"—beginning of insomnia
Problems falling asleep because of stress and anxiety
Frightening dreams
◆ *Adolescence:*
Excessive daytime sleepiness
Extended nocturnal sleep (usually by an hour or more)

Helping your child sleep

Pediatricians and sleep counselors have developed specific guidelines for overcoming your children's sleep problem:

◆ *Develop a pleasant, soothing sleep ritual.* A bedtime story is one of the oldest and most effective. Do not play games that are too stimulating for the children; roughhousing is out of the question.

◆ *Do not arbitrarily decide how much sleep children need at certain ages.* The best way to determine your children's sleep needs is to wake them up at the same time each morning for several days. Notice when they become tired in the evening and what time they went to bed the nights before the mornings when they are especially alert or drowsy. When your children's bodies tell you how much sleep they need, set a bedtime for each child and stick to it.

◆ *Use a neutral device to establish bedtime.* Teach the children where the hands of the clock are at bedtime and have the clock "tell" them when it is time for bed. Or you could use the end of a nightly television show as a signal of bedtime. Do not let bedtime turn into a battle for authority. By relying on an impersonal time-setter, you can avoid considerable conflict.

◆ *Distinguish between bedtime and sleep-time.* Set a definite hour when the children have to get into bed, but do not try to force them to sleep at this time. Let them play quietly with specific bed toys until sleep overtakes them.

◆ *Do not isolate children.* Leave a night-light on; keep the door open; play soft music. These small steps can help lull a child to sleep.

◆ *Be flexible.* Let your children stay up a little later when their friends spend the night. Make an exception to the usual bedtime for a birthday or big holiday.

Typical Daily Sleep Times
(Normal children in familiar surroundings)

AGE	AVERAGE HOURS OF SLEEP
Premature infant (twenty-nine weeks of gestation)	20
Newborn (full forty-week term)	18
Infant (three to nine months)	14
One to two years	13
Two to three years	12
Three to four years	11
Four to five years	10
Six to twelve years	9.5
Twelve to fifteen years	8
Fifteen to nineteen years	7.5

SOURCE: R.L. Williams, I. Karacan, and C.J. Hirsch, *Electroencephalography (EEG) of Human Sleep: Clinical Applications* (New York: John Wiley & Sons, 1974). Reprinted with permission.

But appeal to your children's sense of reason by noting how these late nights make them—like anyone else—sleepier during the day.

♦ *Do not prolong waking.* When you wake up your children in the morning, tell them you are standing by them until they go into the bathroom. Do not allow this time to become a fight for independence.

♦ *Never allow children to sleep in your bed.* This is sure to prolong the normal process of overcoming fears of separation and learning to sleep through the night (see page 263 for guidelines on breaking this habit).

Sleep problems of infancy

Night crying

At the age of two months, 94 percent of babies awaken once or twice in the night; 84 percent of nine-month-old babies continue to awaken. In their first

Making It Through the Night

three years, children are likely to spend an average of nine minutes awake each night.

If your baby wakes up crying, the problem could be physical discomfort, such as an ear infection. Some babies are especially sensitive to travel and new situations and may cry whenever their normal routine is changed. However, if you give your baby too much attention during the night, the problem for both of you is bound to get worse.

Pediatricians realize that parents find it excruciating to listen to a child cry in the night and not do something to provide comfort, but they recommend minimum feedback to the baby between the hours of 10:00 P.M. and 6:00 A.M. If the infant cries every night, eliminate all daytime naps and be sure to put the baby into the crib awake. Move the crib to a separate room if it has been in your bedroom. If the baby cries, wait five minutes before responding. If the crying continues, go into the nursery for no more than one minute to make sure there is no obvious cause of distress. If you must pick the baby up, do so only briefly. If crying persists, check on the baby every thirty minutes for one minute. Again, try not to remove the baby from the crib.

Once your baby has settled into a good sleep pattern, a return to crying at night between the ages of six months and twelve months is a common developmental problem. Approximately 20 percent of babies of this age cry for unexplained reasons during the night. With the development of visual memory, your baby may cry because of separation anxiety. One way to help your baby learn about separation is to play peek-a-boo, providing frequent reassurance that you will return when you are out of sight.

Night feedings

By the age of three months, 70 percent of all babies sleep through the night; by six months, 83 percent are sleeping all night; by one year, 90 percent of babies sleep from dusk to dawn. If your baby is more than four months old and is still insisting—usually by screaming—on night feedings, it is probably because you have trained your baby to expect food around the clock.

This problem is caused by feeding your baby too frequently. You can assure yourself of fewer disturbances in the night if you gradually discontinue all nighttime feedings. Do not allow any bottles in the crib; substitute a pacifier if you must. Schedule the last feeding of the day for 10:00 or 11:00 P.M. The baby should be kept awake while feeding and put to bed awake. The baby's last memory should *not* be of the breast or bottle. If you hear the baby crying in the night, wait one minute before going to the nursery. Hungry babies will not go back to sleep; a slow response will discourage continued awakenings in the night for reasons other than genuine hunger. If you are bottle-feeding your baby, give one ounce less formula than usual at night. Do not breast-feed at night once your baby is past the age of four months. Instead, give formula in a bottle or cup. If you are consistent, the baby will eventually stop wanting food at night.

The problem of night feedings can be prevented by feeding the baby at intervals that are longer than two hours during the day. Give a two-week-old baby a bottle of formula once a week if you are breast-feeding. If you are bottle-feeding, give a bottle of water once a day. Discontinue the 2:00 A.M. feeding when the baby is two months old. Gradually increase the daytime intervals between feedings. Do not use the breast or the bottle as a pacifier. Do not let the baby hold the bottle; make sure the crib is a place for sleeping, not feeding. At night you should go to your baby without waiting and provide reassurance with brief, positive contact. Avoid feeding, and do not hold the baby for more than a few minutes.

SUDDEN INFANT DEATH SYNDROME— "CRIB DEATH"

◆ *Was your baby born prematurely or small for gestational age?*
◆ *Have you ever experienced a "near-miss" episode in which you walked into the nursery to find that your baby had stopped breathing?*

Sudden Infant Death Syndrome (SIDS), or "crib death," is the most common cause of death in infants less than a year old; each year, 10,000 to 18,000 babies die as a result of this problem. Premature or very small babies are most susceptible.

Typically, a seemingly healthy infant, usually one to seven months old, is put to bed according to the daily routine. The baby may have some signs of a

Making It Through the Night

cold or cough. When the parents return to the crib, the child is dead. There is no sign of a struggle, nor does the baby suffocate in the blankets. Autopsies generally reveal, at most, a minor degree of inflammation of the upper respiratory tract or signs of an infectious disease. Determining the cause of death often proves impossible.

Physicians know of no way to predict or prevent crib death. They know more about what does *not* cause SIDS than what does: it is not triggered by external suffocation, vomiting and choking, a contagious disease, bottle-feeding, or hereditary predisposition.

Many physicians believe that a breathing stoppage, or apnea, may be responsible for crib deaths. Central apnea, a disorder of the brain's respiratory control system, may be common in very small and very young infants. For reasons scientists do not yet understand, the brain may fail to direct the movements, or contractions, of the diaphragm during sleep. This may be the result of the immaturity of a newborn's central nervous system. Certainly babies do outgrow the risk of crib death, since this syndrome is rare after seven to twelve months of life.

Some doctors have reported a different type of breathing impairment—obstructive apnea—caused by blockage of the airways. Autopsy has shown that some SIDS victims had mucus plugging their noses. Since children do not learn how to breathe through the mouth until the age of four months, they suffocate if sleeping face-down when the nasal passage is blocked.

Some infants seem to deal with impaired breathing far more easily than others; they cry, flail, and shake when something blocks their normal flow of air. Others are more passive in the same situation and do not initiate the movements that help clear the airway. A lack of oxygen because of obstruction leads to unconsciousness and, within five minutes, death. A psychologist at Brown University, Lewis P. Lipsett, is experimenting with ways to teach small babies to fight for breath. One of his approaches is a sort of peek-a-boo game, in which you put a gauze pad lightly over the infant's nose and mouth, threatening a brief reduction in airflow. A baby who responds by shaking its head and crying is rewarded; others are coaxed to react strongly to the obstruction. Even the youngest infants, he reports, are capable of learning, and though the findings are still preliminary, there does seem to be some hope for teaching all babies how to save their own lives.

SLEEP PROBLEMS OF PRESCHOOLERS

◆ *Does your child fight sleepiness or refuse to go to bed?*
◆ *Does your child seem frightened of the dark?*
◆ *Does your child crawl into your bed at night?*

Researchers believe that sleep problems may be universal in children between the ages of one and five and may be the result of bedtime fears, problems falling asleep, or nightmares and night terrors.

Toddlers need a bedtime ritual, often a complex or repetitive one. Begin by setting a definite bedtime, using the hands of a clock or another impersonal device to indicate that it is time to get ready for bed (see page 257). Teach your children to recognize when the clock indicates that it is bedtime and praise them whenever they realize it on their own. Establish a routine for undressing, washing up, brushing teeth, and getting into pajamas. A bedtime story is one of the nicest of rituals; very young children may find security and comfort in listening to the same story night after night. Allow the children to sleep with a few familiar toys. You may find that children will devise some private sleep rituals. This may include rocking, sucking a thumb or part of the blanket, or masturbating; all are considered normal. Insist that the children get into bed at a regular time, but allow them to play quietly until they are sleepy. Do not deprive them of all stimulation. Leave a soft light on or keep the door open. If they are afraid of the dark or of being alone, reassure them that you will be nearby. These steps can be a formula for improving sleep in toddlers: ritual plus routine plus mother plus toys.

The transition from crib to bed is an important one because a toddler has to leave behind that safe, familiar "friend" of the night. Do not make the change too quickly. Include your child on a shopping trip to buy sheets, bedspread, and a special lamp or clock. Have the child help you make the bed. Decorate a box or carton for bedtime toys and include the old favorites from the crib as well as a few new ones. Follow the same rituals as before, and praise and reward your child for sleeping through the first night in a real bed.

Throughout this period, be wary of providing "secondary gains" in the form of increased attention or pampering to a child who cries at bedtime or during the night. Be careful not to reinforce negative behavior, such as nighttime awakenings. If your child develops a characteristic sleep problem, like waking up frequently, keep a record so you can see whether the problem is getting worse or better. Note your own responses as well as the child's actions.

One of the most trying situations is when children refuse to sleep in their own beds. Often the problem begins when the little boy or girl wakes up crying from a nightmare (page 268) or night terror (page 267) and is carried to the parents' bed. The next night, the scene is replayed—as it is night after night for weeks, or even months. Counselors who have dealt with this situation offer the following guidelines:

1 ◆ Pay attention to your child before bedtime. Read a story. Say prayers together. Tuck the child in. Tell your child that the night should be spent in his or her own bed.

2 ◆ Leave the bedroom door open so the child can hear sounds of other people. If your child is frightened of the dark, leave a night-light on.

3 ◆ If the child sleeps through the night, give praise in the morning.

4 ◆ If your child awakens in the night, go in and provide reassurance. You might sit quietly in the room until the child falls asleep again. However, do not remove the child from the crib or bed.

5 ◆ Be prepared for some difficult nights. Often your child may cry for an hour if not allowed into your bed. Remember that prolonged tears will not harm your child and that sleeping with you may lead to more serious difficulties. By the second and third nights, your child probably will still be crying in the night—but less so. Within a week or two, the problem should be resolved.

ROCKING AND HEAD-BANGING

◆ *Does your child roll his or her head and body before or during sleep?*
◆ *Is your child less than five years old?*
◆ *Are there any daytime signs of emotional, physical, or learning problems?*

"Jactatio capitis nocturnus" is the medical term for rhythmic movements of head or body before or during sleep. Generally this behavior begins before sleep and continues during the early, light stages of NREM sleep. It is common among children under the age of five, occurring in 10 to 30 percent of normal boys and girls and in a higher percentage of children with subnormal intelligence.

The infants of other primates have been observed rocking themselves to sleep, particularly when separated from their mothers. Human children may move their heads and bodies to derive similar comfort. Children usually bang their heads against a headboard or wall or rock to and fro when alone; they may continue this behavior for up to two hours.

This condition usually disappears by adolescence and is considered to be harmless, unless the child also shows neurologic, cognitive, developmental, or emotional abnormalities. Vigorous head-banging, which may seem very violent and alarming to a parent, almost never leads to physical injury. In the absence of any other physical causes, these movements seem related to environmental stress, such as the parents' divorce, the loss of a parent, or pressure to excel in school or sports.

Do not try to stop your child from rocking or banging his or her head in bed; this will only reinforce the behavior. A padded headboard, bed toys, and the presence of familiar, favored playthings—along with a soothing bedtime ritual—may help.

BED-WETTING (ENURESIS)

* *Is your child over five years old and still wetting the bed?*
* *Has your child ever gone through a period of several months without wetting the bed?*
* *Is there a family history of bed-wetting?*

Bed-wetting (enuresis) is the most common childhood sleep problem. It is universal in children less than two years old and in the majority of three-year-olds. By age four, 60 percent of boys and 70 percent of girls are "dry" throughout the night. At age seven, 10 percent of children still wet their beds; some studies suggest that the percentage may actually be higher.

Young children urinate at night because the bladder muscles have not developed sufficiently to control the flow of urine. Children mature at different rates, and boys usually develop this sort of control later than girls. Problems of prolonged enuresis seem to run in families, perhaps because there is a heredi-tary timing to the development of muscle control or because there may be a tendency to have small bladders.

"Primary" enuresis describes children that have never been completely dry for any period of time. This is not considered unusual until age five. "Secondary" enuresis is a recurrence of bed-wetting after a period of dryness. The causes may be emotional, such as the parents' divorce or the arrival of a new baby, or they may be physical causes, including pinworms, infections, breath-ing problems, diabetes, sickle-cell anemia, or disorders of the urinary tract.

Bed-wetting, like night terrors and sleepwalking, is a disorder of partial arousal from deep NREM sleep in the first third of the night. After wetting the bed, the child shifts to lighter sleep. When awakened, the child has no memory of the episode, is unaware of wetting the bed and should not be blamed or scolded. Bed-wetting is a completely involuntary act.

If your child has problems of bed-wetting, be sure to provide reassurance so this physical disorder does not leave psychological scars. Do not get angry or make the child feel ashamed. Most children are acutely embarrassed as it is. They need love and support, not reprimands.

There are many treatment approaches for bed-wetting, varying with the child's age, the frequency of the problem, and the environment. Most physi-cians see no need to "treat" occasional bed-wetting in children at any age. However, you should be sure *not* to reinforce this behavior by taking the child into your bed. Give the child responsibility for washing, changing wet pajamas and bed sheets, and remaking the bed. Keep a calendar by the bed, and put gold stars over each dry night and leave blanks for wet ones. Restrict salty or spicy foods or fluids before bedtime. Older children can be given an alarm clock, set to ring at the time previous episodes have occurred, so they can get up and go to the bathroom before it is too late. Make sure you give them a flashlight or leave some lights on so they can walk to the bathroom without feeling frightened. Or you could provide a bedside urinal.

Occasionally doctors prescribe drugs for bed-wetting. However, the use of drugs is generally limited to keeping a child dry for a specific reason, such as during summer camp. Several behavioral techniques have proved to be effec-tive, including the use of a "bell and pad," in which a bell wakes up the child after wetting. The following is a step-by-step guide to another approach, bladder capacity training:

1 ♦ Once a day have the child retain his or her urine as long as possible before going to the bathroom. Explain that this is the way to learn to hold more and more water in the bladder. The best time for this practice on school days is right after the child comes home.

2 ♦ The child should drink a lot of water, juice, or milk while retaining urine in the bladder. This will help stretch the bladder more quickly.

3 ♦ Using a cup or jar with ounces marked on it, the child should urinate into the cup after holding the urine as long as possible. Have the child measure the number of ounces of urine in the cup.

4 ♦ On a calendar write down the number of ounces of urine produced each day after the urine is retained for as long as possible. Continue to do this every day. Also on the calendar, put a check or gold star on each dry night.

5 ♦ Explain to the child that sometimes it is difficult to hold urine in the bladder for a long time and that it may feel uncomfortable. The child should be kept busy while trying to build up bladder capacity. Try doing something special, like reading or playing games.

6 ♦ After the bladder capacity has increased, have the child practice stopping and starting the urine stream when urinating; this will help develop better control. The child should start doing this just once a day but should soon begin practicing this technique several times a day.

7 ♦ Be patient; both you and your child should see gradual improvement. Keep reinforcing your child's attempts to expand bladder capacity and the ability to sleep through the night without a bed-wetting episode. As dry nights become dry weeks, you might want to give the child a special reward.

SLEEPWALKING (SOMNAMBULISM) SLEEPTALKING (SOMNILOQUY)

♦ *Does your child walk during sleep?*
♦ *Does the child perform simple and repetitive activities during sleep?*
♦ *Does your child talk during sleep?*

Sleepwalking and sleeptalking are common in healthy children. They are disorders of partial arousal from deep NREM sleep and seem to be related to a developmental immaturity in the central nervous system. There also seems to be a familial predisposition to sleepwalking.

Most sleeptalking episodes are brief, and a child rarely says anything intelligible. Sleepwalking generally begins when the child sits up in bed. Usually children walk about, play with their toys, and return to bed. Most episodes last less than thirty minutes; some are longer.

These nighttime activities are *not* signs of emotional or physical disturbances. Try not to focus too much of your attention—or the child's—on nocturnal wanderings. However, do take precautions so that your sleepwalking child is not hurt by falling through a window or down a staircase; barricade all stairways and make sure windows are locked. Keep dangerously sharp objects out of reach. You may want to install a barrier at the child's door.

NIGHT TERRORS (PAVOR NOCTURNUS)

+ *Does your child wake up screaming in the night?*
+ *Does your child breathe rapidly and shallowly and perspire heavily during the awakenings?*
+ *Does your child seem inconsolably upset or frightened?*

Childhood night terrors (pavor nocturnus) are most common in children between the ages of three and seven and seem to be related to abrupt, sudden, incomplete arousal from deep NREM sleep. They occur in at least 3 percent of all children and are not related to emotional disturbances.

The typical attack starts with the child sitting up in bed, yelling, moaning, crying, and speaking incoherently. The child may appear terrified or in pain, with open eyes, deep respiration, rapid heart rate, and heavy perspiration. The child may remain agitated for several minutes to half an hour, often rebuffing a parent that is trying to give comfort. Holding or restraining the child may intensify the outburst.

Often this disorder upsets the parents more than the child. There are obvious signs of physiological distress that the parents can do nothing about. Night terrors seem to be the result of the developmental immaturity of the central nervous system, and in most cases, they disappear by adolescence.

If your child has night terrors, it may be difficult for you to believe that there is nothing seriously wrong. Because your child will not respond to you during the episode, you may become angry and try to rouse him or her fully, usually without success. The best advice is to be available and protective without forcing your attention on your child. As soon as possible, let the child return to sleep.

If these episodes are frequent and disrupt the entire household, consult your pediatrician or a sleep center. In rare circumstances, drugs may be prescribed to prevent night terrors. However, there has been little research on the long-term effects of medications that depress or decrease deep NREM sleep in children.

NIGHTMARES

• *Does your child ever wake up crying and scared, remembering a monster or other phantom in pursuit?*
• *Does your child seem fearful of the bed or of going to sleep?*

Do visions of sugar plums really dance through children's dreams on Christmas Eve? Or are the dreams of the young haunted by fearsome tigers and evil villains?

A dream researcher once described children's nighttime fantasies as "much more complex and much more dreadful than has previously been thought." In his view, the night world of children was a realm of terrors that drove children from their beds to seek the security of their parents' arms. This theory has been challenged and refuted in recent years. Child psychologist Bruno Bettelheim says that children's dreams are "very simple: wishes are fulfilled and anxieties are given tangible form."

Like their elders, children dream as they think about the people, places, and things most familiar to them. A child's mental processes in sleep are no more sophisticated than they are when the child is awake, and children dream about the same sorts of things they talk about during the day. Dream researcher David Foulkes, in his five-year study of the dreams of twenty-six children, developed the following chronology of dream topics and themes:

AGE THREE TO FOUR Children have very simple dreams; the characters tend to be animals rather than people. The action is performed by the rabbits or chickens, not by the dreamer, and is quite mundane, like eating or drinking.

AGES THREE TO FOUR: Children have very simple dreams; the characters tend to be animals rather than people. The action is performed by the rabbits or chickens, not by the dreamer, and is quite mundane, like eating or drinking.

AGES FIVE TO SIX: Dreams become twice as long by this age, and there is conflict.

AGES SEVEN TO EIGHT: Dreams become fairly complex, with plots and subplots. The content is highly personal and reflects the child's wish to become a competent adult. Boys now dream more about family and friends and less about animals or fighting.

AGES THIRTEEN TO FOURTEEN: At this age, dreams become more obscure and complex. Girls dream more about women; boy's dreams have more aggressive themes. Both have dreams with vague settings and enigmatic meanings.

Dream researcher Rosalind Cartwright categorizes children's dreams according to whether the cause, or "agency," is bad or good and inside or outside the dreamer. "Bad outside" dreams begin earliest, usually at ages five to twelve; "good-due-to-own-efforts" dreams predominate from ages nine to twelve; "bad-due-to-personal inadequacy" dreams come later, around age fifteen.

Children's scary dreams fall in four basic categories, according to Cartwright's theory: those concerning physical sensations, those with psychological components, social interaction dreams, and strange or supernatural dreams. Children that are younger than ten usually have aggression dreams in which they are threatened by an animal or monster. Adolescents dream of psychological anxiety, such as being in competition or in a socially embarrassing situation.

Children probably do not have bad dreams more often than adults, but they tend to remember the more dramatic and upsetting scenes. Children's dreams are particularly frightening because they may not be able to distinguish them from reality and may not have the vocabulary to express their feelings and fears.

You can help your children deal with scary dreams by encouraging them to talk about their nighttime fantasies. Explain that having a dream is like telling a story to oneself. The dreamer, as "writer" or "storyteller," can change the dream in any way. If your child tells you of being chased by a bear in a dream, have the child think of a way to get out of danger—by climbing a tree, or perhaps by shooting the bear. Encourage the child to use this solution if the dream recurs. If your child has some sense of control over the creatures of dreams, sleep will seem much less scary and mysterious.

Talking about dreams can also be a good way to find out what your child is thinking or feeling troubled about. You might use the dream reports to launch discussions of how your child feels about a planned move, a conflict between two parents, or about difficulties in school.

TOOTH-GRINDING (BRUXISM)

• *Does your child clench his or her teeth or grind them during sleep?*
• *Has the family dentist commented on abnormal wear patterns on your child's teeth?*

Children, like many adults, may gnash and grind their teeth during the night. Sleep researchers estimate that 15 percent of normal, healthy boys and girls are "nocturnal bruxists." Children rarely know that they are grinding their teeth during sleep, but the sounds they make may be audible in other rooms.

Bruxism seems to occur intermittently, generally in Stage 2 of NREM sleep. There seems to be no relationship to dream content in REM periods, and scientists believe it may be caused by many factors, including stress, personality characteristics, genetic predisposition, elongated teeth, poor fillings, and malocclusion of the upper and lower teeth (see page 195 for information on adult bruxism). Sometimes the problem decreases after childhood.

Proper dental care may eliminate the problem. Occasionally, "night guards," or bite plates, are recommended to prevent damage to teeth, gums,

Making It Through the Night

and mouth muscles. For adults, a variety of behavioral techniques have proved to be effective, but there has not been similar success with children.

BREATHING PROBLEMS (SLEEP APNEA)

♦ *Does your child snore loudly?*
♦ *Are there pauses or silences between gasping, choking sounds?*
♦ *Does your school-age child wet the bed? Has your child started to wet the bed after years of dryness?*

An apnea is a temporary breathing stoppage, caused either by a blockage of the upper airway (obstructive apnea) or by an impaired respiratory control system in the brain (central apnea). Sleep apnea seems to play a major role in Sudden Infant Death Syndrome (see page 260). Apnea has not been studied or diagnosed extensively in children, but adults with apnea report that their symptoms often started before the age of sixteen.

More than 90 percent of apnea victims are males. In children, obstructive apnea is more common, and the cause is likely to be anatomical, such as enlarged tonsils and adenoids or excessive fatty tissue in the airway. The clue to this disorder is extremely loud snoring, usually increasing gradually over several months or years. Virtually all children with apnea wet their beds. More than half of older children with apnea have early morning headaches and elevated blood pressure; many are overweight.

Childhood apnea can lead to the development of chronic, ultimately life-threatening illnesses, such as heart disease and cardiac arrhythmias. It also can have devastating mental and emotional side effects. Chronic oxygen shortages may impair intellectual development and learning ability. Even when the child's intelligence is not impaired, he or she may be labeled as retarded or lazy because of excessive sleepiness. Such children may have many behavior problems, including hyperactivity, as they try to keep themselves awake by constant motion. Bizarre, frightening hallucinations may occur as the children are falling asleep, making them frightened of going to bed at night.

Often the solution to childhood sleep apnea is remarkably simple: removal of the enlarged tonsils and adenoids. In more complicated or severe cases, a tracheostomy—a surgical opening into the windpipe to allow passage of air—may be performed. Since the air tube into the throat is covered during the day, the child can continue normal daytime activities, including sports. Drug therapy is rarely attempted in children. (For more information about sleep apnea, see pages 192 and 227.)

CHILDHOOD INSOMNIA

◆ *Does your child complain of not being able to sleep at night?*
◆ *Has your child recently been ill or hospitalized?*
◆ *Is it a time of family trauma?*
◆ *Is your child having problems at school?*

Young children may insist that they will not go to sleep and refuse to get into bed, stay in bed, or stop crying. Older children and adolescents sound more like grown-ups when they complain that, try as they may, they cannot sleep.

Researchers once thought that childhood insomnia was a rarity. However, a surprisingly high percentage of adults with chronic sleep problems trace their origins back to their childhood. Some children definitely seem to live by a different time clock. They are the ones who never take afternoon naps, sneak toys or books into their beds at night, and do not willingly get out of bed in the morning. Like adults, others have medical problems that keep them awake at night: pains, itches, indigestion, splints for broken bones, allergies, and many childhood diseases.

Very often the reason a child cannot sleep is emotional rather than physiological. Stress is just as real in a child's world as it is for adults, although it takes different forms: pressures to do well in school, trying to make an athletic team, feeling snubbed by a group of classmates, anxiety about parental divorce or separation, birth of siblings, a move to a strange place, death of a beloved pet. Since these are situational problems, they usually resolve themselves in time. If your child's sleeplessness persists for more than six weeks, you should consider psychological care.

In a very small number of instances, childhood-onset insomnia may be caused by disorders of the brain's sleep controls that are too subtle to be detected by current methods. Sleeplessness is likely to plague these people for the nights of their lives, and no remedy yet devised offers help or hope. By adulthood, the lack of rest may lead to total disability, psychological problems, and an unusual sensitivity to any drugs that act on the brain.

NARCOLEPSY

♦ *Does your child seem quite sleepy during the day?*
♦ *Does your child seem to be in perpetual motion at times, refusing to stay still for any period of time?*
♦ *Have your child's teachers reported any behavioral problems to you?*
♦ *Does your school-age child still wet the bed?*

Narcolepsy, a disorder of the mechanisms of sleep and wakefulness, is considered rare in children (for a complete description of narcolepsy, see page 222 to 227). However, its symptoms often may not be recognized. A sleepy child may try to counter drowsiness by running, rolling, and staying in motion; some adult narcoleptics recall that they were considered "hyperactive" as children. Teachers may think that a child who dozes off briefly in class is lazy or uninterested or has a learning problem. Sometimes other sleep disorders may be a clue that your child has narcolepsy. Ten percent of narcoleptics who were diagnosed by age sixteen said that they wet the bed until age ten; 18 percent said they were frequent sleepwalkers.

Since narcolepsy is a progressive disease, other symptoms—such as muscle weakness (cataplexy), disturbed nighttime sleep, bizarre hallucinations, and sleep paralysis on awakening—may not occur in children. However, the children are likely to have peculiar daytime behavior, including long naps, and may be fearful of going to sleep because of the extraordinarily vivid hallucinations they have while falling asleep and waking up. Half of all narcoleptics report that at least one of their major symptoms developed before the age of sixteen.

If you are a narcoleptic, your child is much more likely to develop narcolepsy than other children. If you suspect narcolepsy, have your child evaluated at a sleep center. Sleep recordings (see page 288) will confirm the diagnosis by determining whether or not the child begins REM sleep almost immediately after falling asleep.

Most physicians are reluctant to give children the drugs that have become standard for adults because their long-range effects are unknown. However, proper diagnosis can ensure that the child is not labeled as hyperactive or mentally retarded and can help the family plan a schedule that allows for daytime naps.

CHAPTER 18

Going Gently Into the Night:
Sleep Problems of the Elderly

Y ou may think of the last decades of your life as a time for well-earned rest after years of toil. But the older you are, the less time you sleep each night—and the more likely you are to complain about sleep problems.

Normal, healthy eighty-year-olds spend one-fifth of the night awake. It takes them eighteen minutes to fall asleep, and total sleep time amounts to six hours. Only a few minutes—if any time at all—are spent in the deepest type of sleep, NREM Stage 4, and a little more than an hour in REM sleep. They probably take at least one nap a day.

Compare this sleep pattern to the way things were at age twenty: Twenty-year-olds fall asleep in 8 minutes, spend 95 percent of the night asleep, sink into deep NREM sleep for half an hour or more and dream for almost 2 hours of the night. Their total sleep time averages 7.5 to 8 hours, and they do not nap during the day.

The nights of your life change as dramatically as your days as you grow older. But they tend to change gradually, almost imperceptibly over time. Sleep cycles do not take on a new pattern when you retire or become seventy years old; they are evolving from the moment of birth. A child of ten sleeps half as much as a newborn and spends 30 percent less time in REM at night. A thirty-year-old spends half as much time as a twenty-year-old in deep Stage 4 sleep and wakes up twice as often in the night. Men start sleeping lighter and for less time in their thirties; women's sleep changes most after menopause.

At any age the quality of sleep is always a subjective appraisal. In most surveys 15 percent of adults complain that they do not sleep well; by age seventy, 30 percent express concern over their sleep. Older women report many more sleep problems than men. In both sexes, the primary worries are problems falling asleep, frequent awakenings in the night, early morning awakenings, and daytime sleepiness.

Not all people over the age of sixty sleep poorly; most do *not* say that they have sleep problems. The quality of sleep reflects the quality of health, mood, and satisfaction with life, and vice-versa. Researchers have found that older men and women who sleep as they did in previous years—particularly if they spend as much time in REM sleep as before—have fewer changes in their mental functioning.

You should expect some differences in your sleep as you grow older, just as you expect—even if you do not eagerly await—such transformations as gray hair and wrinkled skin. At seventy, you do not look like the twenty-year-old you once were, and you cannot expect to sleep the way you did then. Sometimes elderly people think of their changed sleep patterns at ages sixty and seventy as serious problems rather than the normal consequences of aging. However, sometimes shortened, fragmented sleep—particularly if it develops rather quickly—may be a sign of a serious physical or psychological disturbance. An understanding of the sleep patterns that are common after age sixty may reassure you or alert you to seek help for an actual sleep disorder.

Normal aging

Sleep changes in four basic ways during one's life: less total sleep time, much less deep NREM sleep, a little less REM sleep, and more waking periods in the night. The solid sleep of childhood and young adulthood gradually becomes lighter and more fragmented. REM sleep occurs much earlier in the night. In extreme old age, the sleeper seems unable to consolidate sleep into long periods and tends to sleep, much like a newborn does, in snatches or naps around the clock. These changes occur in all types of elderly people—in one researcher's phrase, to the "rich and poor, able and infirm, nice and nasty."

Since sleep is a change in consciousness—a state of mind—it reflects changes in our organ of consciousness, the brain. As the brain ages, sleep changes. Over a seventy or eighty-year period, 20 percent of the brain's nerve cells (neurons) cease to function. For unknown reasons, more neurons stop functioning during our forties than in the years before or after.

The brain shows other signs of slow degeneration: decreased blood flow and increased senile plaques (areas of partial tissue death) in the brain. There is also a gradual lowering of the background frequency of brain waves while awake, from ten to twelve cycles per second in youth to eight to ten cycles per second in old age. This reflects the brain's functional state. The higher the background frequency, the more alert you are likely to be. On studies of older people, those with the lowest brain wave frequencies were less alert and less able to learn a new verbal performance skill. At night, those with higher alertness and brain wave frequencies had more REM sleep, while senile persons had much less REM.

These degenerative changes in the brain and nervous system—seemingly beyond our control—may be responsible for the changes in sleep with age and the variations in different individuals. In general, the more alert you are when awake, the better you are likely to sleep.

Sleep researcher Irwin Feinberg, M.D., of the Veterans Administration Medical Center in San Francisco has found that changed sleep patterns in the elderly are related to impaired memory. He feels this is an indication that the brain's ability to process information is indeed related to sleep. Perhaps sleep-time declines because, with age, we need to process less information. As the intensity of brain activity lessens, so does the amount of restoration required of sleep.

Rhythm changes

Dozens of your basic physiological functions are coordinated and timed by your biological clock, which sets the rhythms for the days, months and years of your life (see chapter 2, "Sunrise, Sunset," page 213). Could your internal clock simply slow down with age? There is evidence that this does indeed happen. In one study where subjects were isolated from time cues, all of those between the ages of forty-four and sixty-nine became "desynchronized," while only 21 percent of the younger subjects developed rhythm problems. The older you are, the more you will suffer from jet lag (page 241) or changes in work shift (page 239), possibly because your internal time-setter grows weaker. Perhaps the ability of different organ systems to work in harmony diminishes with age, or there may be a decline in the powers of your internal rhythm regulators. In studying "circa-annual," or yearly, rhythms, researchers have noted significant changes with each decade of life.

The sleep-wake cycle is one of the most important rhythms of life, and it may reflect the degenerative changes in your body clock. External factors may also influence the sleep-wake cycle. The strongest human "zeitgeber," or pacesetter, is the stimulation of other people. An older person who retires from work, lives alone, and keeps an erratic schedule may not have the social cues to maintain a rhythm. In nursing homes or hospitals, the elderly live formless lives, resting and sleeping at irregular times of day as well as night. The lack of a strong rhythm and routine in the environment can make it impossible for their internal clockworks, already depressed by age, to preserve harmony and health.

If you are retired and can set your own hours, establish a daily routine. Always get up at the same time, and eat your meals at the same hours of the day. If possible, try not to live in isolation. Companionship and outside interests can add great satisfaction, as well as structure, to the hours of your day. While most people feel an increasing need to nap as they grow older, do not spend too much time in bed during the day because this may make it more difficult for you to consolidate your sleep into a long period at night.

Medical problems

Your sleep may be affected by anything that ails you during the day. Some diseases that are common or severe in the elderly, such as arthritis, may be especially disruptive at night. The pain caused by body movements during sleep is one of the most common reasons why older people awaken in the night. (The section on medical problems in chapter 16, page 243 describes some of the other physical disorders that disrupt sleep.) If you have had an illness or injury or have a chronic medical problem, ask your doctor about its possible effect on your sleep. Be especially careful about the medications you take, because any drug that acts on the mind can influence sleep. Changes in dosage or timing of an essential remedy may help you rest more easily.

At any age, regular physical activity enhances the quality of sleep; remain as active as you can. Gentle stretching exercises may be especially soothing before bedtime. Avoid stimulating substances like cigarettes and coffee; their sleep-disrupting effects increase greatly in the elderly, even among volunteers who believed that caffeine could not affect their sleep.

Psychological factors

The "golden years" after retirement may be tarnished by the loss of a beloved spouse or close friends, by worry about health or finances, by loneliness, and by the loss of the self-esteem and gratifications provided by rewarding jobs. Your sleep may be the best mirror of these changes. Anticipation, anxiety, depression, and fear can keep a person of any age awake at night. The older you are, the more sensitive your sleep may be to the feelings you experience during the day. You may not be conscious of the "hidden" factors affecting your sleep, or you may find it difficult to talk about your emotions or seek help in coping with your feelings and fears.

Sometimes the "leisure" you looked forward to after retirement turns out to be less relaxing and more tedious than anticipated. Some psychologists feel that "old-age boredom" can be a hidden reason for complaints of insomnia. Stay active in mind and body, enjoy the company of others, and remain interested in the world around you, and you may sleep better at night.

The psychological challenges of aging are complex. The only easy advice is to avoid easy answers. There is a tendency, on the part of physicians as well as patients, to prescribe or use medications rather than address the real problems. Talking about your feelings and expressing bottled-up emotions are good ways to begin coping with the challenge of aging.

Use of sleeping pills

In 1974, individuals over the age of sixty-four constituted 15 percent of the American population but consumed 33 percent of the prescription sleeping pills used that year. In one group of women over age seventy-five, 45 percent used sleeping pills regularly; a survey in the San Francisco area found that 48 percent of adults over the age of sixty-five used a sleep aid often. The rates for sleeping pill use in nursing homes and hospitals are even higher. Ironically, the overuse of sleeping pills results in *less* sleep and more sleep problems in the elderly.

Part of the reason older people use so many sleeping pills is that they tend to use more of all kinds of drugs. There are 11.4 prescriptions written each year for each person over sixty-five, as compared to 4 for each younger adult. This high drug use is dangerous because there can be fatal interactions of drugs in the body, particularly in combination with sleeping pills.

As is explained in chapter 10, "The Perils of Sleeping Pills," no sleeping pill provides a lasting solution to the problem of sleeplessness. Many pills lead to physical and psychological dependence and create lingering side-effects. These problems are much more serious in elderly persons, who may not metabolize and excrete drugs as quickly as younger individuals. A drug that remains in the body of a thirty-year old for twenty-four hours may be found in the blood of a seventy-year old days after it was ingested. The reasons for this retention include a lower percentage of fatty tissue to absorb certain drugs, fewer intestinal cells for absorption, decreased intestinal blood flow, diminished ability of the liver to metabolize drugs, and greatly lessened blood flow through the kidney, impairing the body's ability to excrete drugs. If you take a nightly sleeping pill, you are adding to the build-up of medications in your body.

Sleeping pills are usually tested on young, healthy adults, and physicians do not know the special risks to the elderly. They have observed that frequent use of sleep aids lessens deep sleep and increases awakening in the night. Mood and daytime performance may be impaired. Some aged patients become agitated or confused as a result of chronic use of sleeping pills, particularly if they show other signs of brain degeneration. Often these episodes are treated with more sedatives. Oversedation of the elderly has led to a major public health problem. In one study, a sixth of the older patients that were admitted to mental hospitals "recovered" completely once they were withdrawn from sedatives and sleeping pills.

Doctors have been criticized for "pushing pills" on elderly patients rather than spending the necessary time to help them resolve difficult emotional issues. However, many elderly patients prefer and even demand chemical solutions and start using over-the-counter drugs if their physicians refuse to give them prescription sleeping pills. Sometimes financial factors play a role. Living on fixed incomes, the aged may prefer an inexpensive sleep aid because it costs less money than a visit to the doctor. Lack of transportation or physical impairments may make it extremely inconvenient for them to visit a physician for a problem that they perceive as "simple," such as sleeplessness.

In its report on sleeping pill use in the United States, the National Academy of Sciences listed "common and potentially dangerous self-medication behaviors" in the elderly: "lack of knowledge of what constitutes a side-effect; taking medications irregularly because of lack of motivation; forgetfulness, expense or self-determination of need; borrowing and lending medicines; saving old medications and using them to self-treat problems; mixing different drugs in one container; overdosage by ingestion of duplicate medications prescribed by different physicians."

There are other dangers that can prove fatal. Sleep apnea is more common in older persons, and sleeping pills may interfere with the brain's signals to the body to resume respiration (see pages 192 and 227 for an explanation of apnea and how it can be treated). Older people who take pills often wake up confused in the middle of the night; this disorientation may be the cause of falls and injuries. The ingredients in many sleeping pills may cause complications in people with high blood pressure, heart disease, and other chronic medical impairments.

The National Academy of Science urged physicians to be conservative in prescribing sleeping pills for elderly patients and to prescribe only the lowest possible doses. Dalmane (flurazepam), the most popular sleeping pill in the country, should be given to older people only in doses that are half the usual amount because this substance stays in the body for an extremely long period.

Adverse effects of sleeping pills may be quite different in the elderly and may include intoxication, an alarming drop in blood pressure, restlessness, and aggression. Even sleeping pills that rarely produce side-effects in younger patients may lead to serious physical and psychological complications in older users, including visual hallucinations, memory loss, and coordination problems. They also may mask a serious underlying problem, such as deep depression that could lead to a suicide attempt.

A better night's sleep

If you are over sixty years old, you cannot expect to sleep like a kid again. However, you can help yourself sleep better. The first step, if you have been taking sleeping pills for a long period of time, is to see your physician. With close medical supervision, begin gradual withdrawal. You may have a few restless nights, but if you slowly wean yourself from the drugs, you will eventually restore your body's natural sleep-wake rhythm.

Just as you may change your life-style because of retirement or advancing age, you should plan on some adjustments in your sleep style. Develop a long, soothing nighttime ritual. Gerontologist Robert Butler, M.D., and his colleagues recommend soaking in a warm tub, back massage, wine, warm sake (Japanese rice wine) and pleasurable sexual activity, including masturbation.

Set up a schedule for your daytime activity with definite times for rising, meals, chores, and other activities. Reduce your napping in the daytime. Try not to go to bed too early. If you wake up at a definite time each day and let your body determine its best sleep time at night, you'll probably wake up less often during the night.

Take care of your health: eat nutritious, light meals; try to get some daily exercise. You may find that exercise gives you more daytime energy as well as helping you to sleep at night. Reduce your use of stimulants such as cigarettes and coffee.

If you fill your days with activities that interest and please you, your nights may also become more satisfying. Retirement is the time to begin a hobby that you have postponed for decades because of work pressures. Reach out to others. Many older people withdraw into an ever-shrinking world, sometimes because of physical disability, sometimes because of the loss of familiar friends and loved ones. Humans are social creatures at all ages. The company of others is a timeless, ageless joy.

CHAPTER 19

Sleep Centers

S leep medicine is one of the newest of medical specialities. Two decades ago there were a few interested researchers but no special facilities for people with sleep problems. Now there are dozens of specialized sleep programs in operation around the country (see page 291 for a complete list). In 1976 the Association of Sleep Disorders Centers was organized to set standards and act as the certifying body for these facilities and their staffs.

Not all sleep clinics are alike. They may be sponsored by psychiatry, neurology, or internal medicine departments. Relatively few are designed to serve as regional referral centers. Most have fewer than six beds; many are housed within hospitals; some share equipment with neurology departments. The larger clinics are affiliated with major medical centers and call upon the specialized expertise of a variety of physicians, including internists, neurologists, psychiatrists, cardiologists, and others. The smaller centers may refer certain patients to larger centers for specific treatments.

Every major sleep center has the sophisticated equipment needed to perform "polysomnograms"—night-long recordings of various physiological functions. Specially trained technicians are responsible for the maintenance of these machines and for the all-night monitorings; a physician is always on call during such tests. Some sleep therapists undergo rigorous testing for certification as "clinical polysomnographers." These experts, who must be medical doctors or health professionals with doctoral degrees, interpret the nightly recordings to determine a diagnosis.

Should you go to a sleep center?

A sleep center is usually not the first place to go for help with a sleep problem. Many people can recognize and remedy their sleep problems on their own because they are the result of rather straightforward factors, such as irregular schedules or overuse of stimulants. The questionnaires in chapter 11 (page 160) should give you a better understanding of what may be keeping you awake at night. If the underlying problem is tension, you can try relaxation therapies (see page 113). If there seems to be a medical disorder or if your self-care remedies fail to work, you should see a physician. Your doctor will try to rule out any physical ailments that might be disturbing your sleep. If you are going through a difficult period in your life, if you are older and worried about your changing sleep pattern, or if you normally sleep few hours, your doctor might reassure you that your sleep "difficulty" is not a reason for worry.

Sleep medicine is so new that most physicians have received little, if any, training in it. Only recently have medical schools begun to include at least a few lectures on sleep in their curricula, and a federally supported program, Project Sleep, is educating more practicing doctors about sleep disorders. If you have had a sleep problem for several months, your physician may refer you to a sleep center.

Many people with excessive daytime sleepiness have consulted doctors for years without finding help. The two most serious causes of daytime tiredness—narcolepsy (page 222) and obstructive sleep apnea (page 227)—have been extensively studied by sleep specialists only in recent years. If your symptoms match those described in the sections on these disorders, you may want to contact a sleep center in your area directly. Or you could ask your doctor to refer you to the center.

Ultimately you are the best judge of whether or not you should be evaluated at a sleep center. If your sleep problem is interfering with your daytime functioning and mood, if it is chronic and severe rather than occasional, you should turn to a sleep center for help.

What should you expect?

Sleep centers are designed to provide an accurate, highly specific diagnosis of your problem. First, you will be asked to fill out extensive questionnaires (the questionnaires in chapter 11, page 160, will prepare you for the types of questions you will be asked). In addition, you will be given a complete physical exam and a battery of psychological tests, including an inventory of recent life changes, tests of personality, interest, and preference, and a sophisticated test to measure behavior patterns that indicate emotional disturbance. You will also be asked for an extensive medical history, including details of the history of your sleep complaints, your mental and physical health, your family's health and sleep habits, and your personal life (including use of drugs, relationships, career, money, sexual problems, and so on). At some centers, you may be questioned by a psychologist or psychiatrist about emotional aspects of your sleep problem, such as what you think about when you are lying awake, whether you associate the bedroom with any trauma, whether you fear falling asleep, and so on. A neurologist will evaluate your perceptual skills and your ability to react quickly and correctly to various stimuli. Other tests include analysis of a urine specimen, blood test, and blood pressure reading. You will be asked to keep a sleep log; you may also be requested to live by a very regular timetable for the next few weeks and to fill out a daytime sleepiness scale. If you have been taking sleeping pills, your doctor may want to withdraw you from them before scheduling an all-night sleep recording.

Sometimes this information is sufficient for specialists to make a diagnosis. For example, if the tests show that you are depressed, you will be referred for treatment to help your daytime mood and functioning so that your nighttime sleep can also improve. If you have a nutritional deficiency or a medical condition, you will be directed to physicians who can treat these problems. Sometimes your sleep history alone—for example, years of waking up screaming in the night—will pinpoint exactly what the problem is (night terrors, in this case). In cases of chronic and severe sleeplessness or sleepiness, the sleep therapists will recommend an all-night sleep recording to find out exactly what is happening to you during the night. This sort of evaluation may be essential for correct diagnosis of a problem and determination of how severe it is.

If your problem is excessive daytime sleepiness, you might be evaluated by a daytime procedure called a Multiple Sleep Latency Test (MSLT). At two-hour periods throughout the day, you are hooked up to a polysomnograph before taking a brief nap. Your tendency to fall asleep quickly and your entry into REM sleep may confirm a diagnosis of narcolepsy.

Electrodes are attached to patient's face and head in preparation for night of study in the sleep laboratory. Courtesy Adrian N. Bouchard, Dartmouth College.

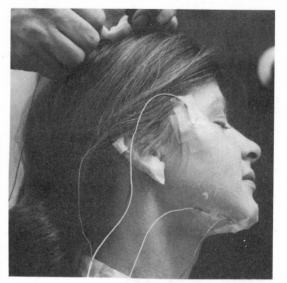

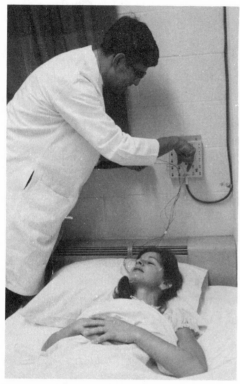

As the patient settles in for a night in the sleep lab, a sleep researcher attaches electrodes from the patient to the central line of polysomnographic equipment. Courtesy Adrian N. Bouchard, Dartmouth College.

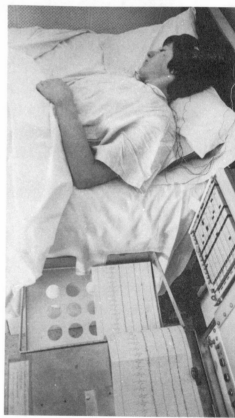

Patient sleeps soundly as equipment monitors her sleeping patterns and activity. Courtesy Milton Kramer, M.D., and Thomas Roth, Ph.D.

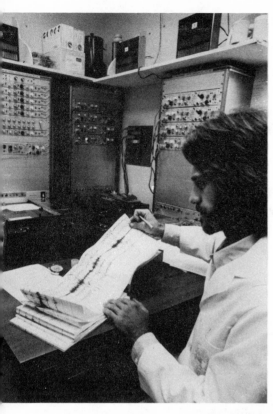

Courtesy Milton Kramer, M.D., and
Thomas Roth, Ph.D.

A sleep researcher studies all-night sleep
recordings and close-up, below.

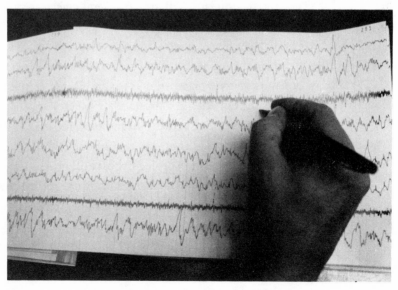

Courtesy
Adrian N. Bouchard,
Dartmouth College.

What is involved in an all-night sleep recording?

An all-night sleep recording is a way of monitoring brain waves, heart rhythm, respiration, temperature, and body movement through the night. Although it involves equipment used in other medical tests (such as an EEG machine), it is unlike most medical evaluations. First of all, you sleep right through it. There is no pain or discomfort, other than the slight initial irritation of the electrodes. There are no injections, no anesthetics, no incisions, no X rays. All that is required of you is to sleep as you usually do. If you are afraid that you will not be able to fall asleep in the unfamiliar setting, be assured that many patients have felt the same way. Sleep specialists have learned how to recognize and discount the "first-nighter" effects.

You will be told to come to the sleep center late in the evening, not too many hours before your usual bedtime. Most of the sleep settings look like a cross between a motel and a hospital room; they are not luxurious, but they are comfortable, quiet, and dark. An intercom will allow you to speak to the technician at any time of the night. In some cases, your sleep may be filmed by an infrared camera; this visual information is important in recording the unusual body movements associated with specific sleep disorders.

You will change into pajamas or nightgown at the center. If you want, bring your own pillow and your usual nighttime reading. After you are dressed for sleep, the technicians will attach several electrodes to your face and body. These are placed *on* the skin, usually over an ointment that is dabbed on to form a better seal; they are *not* injected like needles. All are arranged in pairs so if one falls off during the night, the other serves as backup. Two are placed on the chin to record muscle tone or tension. Two are placed at the corner of the eyes to measure eye movement. A "ground" is placed on the forehead to prevent ambient electromagnetic activity from being recorded. Two are placed on the top of the scalp to detect brain waves. Other electrodes on the upper right and lower left of the chest measure heartbeats. Temperature-sensitive devices are taped under the nostrils and at the mouth; these record the breath rate and the volume of inhaled air. An electrode on each leg records leg movements before or during sleep. A beltlike gadget around the lower chest monitors the movements of the diaphragm. If sleep apnea is suspected, a small microphone may be placed beneath the nose to allow the technician to listen to your breathing. You also may be asked a few questions about your presleep thoughts and feelings.

The electrodes do not hurt, but initially they may be distracting, like insects that have landed on your face. When you get into bed, the electrodes will be hooked up to the central line of the polysomnograph equipment. Although the wires are firmly secured, they are not confining. You will be able to sit up, turn to either side, and, usually with the technician's help in "unplugging" yourself, get up and go to the bathroom.

The technician will make note of the time you turn out the lights and, by watching the brain waves recorded on the polysomnograph, when you fall asleep. All night long the electrodes will send signals to the polysomnograph; these are converted into electrical impulses that appear as wavy lines on the continuous sheets of paper fed into the machine. During the sleep recording of one night, more than half a mile of paper may be covered with squiggles and waves.

In the morning you will be asked to answer questions about how you slept, including estimates of how long it took for you to fall asleep, how often you awakened, and how this night compared to a "normal" night's sleep. The data from the polysomnograph is usually processed by computer, which calculates actual sleep latency, time in each sleep stage, awakenings, breathing stoppages, changes in heart rate, and final awakening. A trained polysomnographer will assess these data to make a diagnosis. In some cases, you may be asked to spend more than one night in the laboratory to supply further information on how you sleep.

What is the cost of a sleep center's services?

The diagnostic workup for a sleep disorder is not cheap. A typical sleep center might charge $170 or more for initial evaluation (history, physical examinations, interviews, lab tests, psychological assessment); and $400 to $800 for all-night sleep recordings. There are additional charges for each subsequent polysomnogram and visits and for consultations with various specialists.

The charges reflect the high cost of equipment and staff time. Sleep specialists feel that the benefits are worth the cost if the patient finds the answer to the disorder that has been disturbing nighttime sleep and daytime functioning. However, they note that cost-benefit equation balances only for those patients who have serious, chronic problems, not for those with occasional complaints of sleeplessness.

Your insurance company may or may not pay for polysomnography, depending on the nature and severity of your problem. The most comprehensive health plans, including those provided by Blue Cross, will cover diagnostic tests for sleep disorders because they are laboratory tests. The need for these tests is clear-cut in such serious disorders as narcolepsy or obstructive apnea, which may require surgery (a tracheostomy). Some companies, however, do not provide coverage for insomnia workups. If you have questions about your policy, check with your insurance agent. Medicare and Medicaid generally will cover specific services of a sleep center.

Will you find a way to sleep better?

There are no guarantees in sleep medicine—or any other field of medicine. However, the directors of sleep centers are optimistic about their ability to help people who have been troubled sleepers for years. Generally, they estimate their success rate to be about 75 to 80 percent, but there is enormous variation in different types of patients. If the underlying problem is depression, more than 90 percent of patients can be helped. The improvements in apnea patients depend on the treatment suggested and agreed upon. For people with drug-caused insomnia, withdrawal is a virtually universal cure. Chronotherapy has proved to be helpful for most people with desynchronized body clocks. The estimates of improvement in those with chronic anxiety or tension are not as high—perhaps 60 to 70 percent. The patient's motivation is the key to real improvement in the sleep disorders that arise from the mind as well as the body.

The major sleep centers usually follow up their patients to check on progress and problems. However, because they are referral rather than treatment centers, they may refer you back to the care of your own physician once the diagnosis has been made and treatment has been initiated.

Are there less expensive alternatives?

A major technological advance in sleep medicine has been the development of portable equipment to allow home sleep recordings. One unit contains the necessary equipment in a briefcase-sized carrier and relays the signals to the laboratory via telephone. Manufacturers are also developing sensitive monitors that can be worn twenty-four hours a day to measure heart and respiratory activity. Such ambulatory monitoring can provide critical information in patients with suspected heart disease. A much simpler wristwatch-sized device is also available and can supply a record of periods of activity and of rest.

This equipment, available at only a few sleep centers and appropriate for only some patients, is important because it may reduce the cost of sleep evaluation. The current fees range from $50 to $250. Eventually, the sleep specialists say, all of us might use monitoring devices as part of a regular "sleep physical," a checkup of a nighttime well-being.

You should keep in mind that a sleep evaluation may be as vital to your well-being as any other medical test. The benefits of identifying a chronic sleep problem and learning a way to correct or cope with it can be priceless.

How can you find a sleep center near you?

The following list of sleep centers was provided by the Association of Sleep Disorders Centers:

Sleep Disorders Center
Holy Cross Hospital
15031 Rinaldi Street
Mission Hills, CA 91345
Attn: Elliott R. Phillips

Sleep Disorders Center
U.C. Irvine Medical Center
101 City Drive South
Orange, CA 92688
Attn: Jon Sassin, M.D.

Sleep Disorders Program
Stanford University Med. Center
Stanford, CA 94305
Attn: Laughton Miles, M.D.

Sleep Disorders Center
Mt. Sinai Medical Center
4300 Alton Road
Miami Beach, FL 33140
Attn: Martin A. Cohn, M.D.

Sleep Disorders Center
Northwestern Memorial Hospital
250 E. Superior Street
Chicago, IL 60611
Attn: Juan J. Cayaffa, M.D.

Sleep Disorders Center
Rush-Presbyterian-St. Luke's
1753 W. Congress Parkway
Chicago, IL 60612
Attn: Rosalind Cartwright, Ph.D.

Sleep Disorders Center
Psychiatry and Neurology
Tulane Medical School
New Orleans, LA 70118
Attn: John Goeth, M.D.

Sleep Disorders Center
Department of Neurology
Univ. of Mass. Med. Center
Worcester, MA 01605
Attn: Sheldon Kapen, M.D.

Sleep Disorders Center
Baltimore City Hospital
Baltimore, MD 21224
Attn: Richard Allen, Ph.D.

Sleep Disorders Center
Henry Ford Hospital
2799 W. Grand Blvd.
Detroit, MI 48202
Attn: Thomas Roth, Ph.D.

Sleep Disorders Center
Neurology Department
Hennepin Co. Med. Center
Minneapolis, MN 55415
Attn: Milton Ettinger, M.D.

Sleep Disorders Center
Department of Psychiatry
Dartmouth Medical School
Hanover, NH 03755
Attn: Michael Sateia, M.D.

Sleep-Wake Disorders Center
Montefiore Hospital
111 E. 210th Street
Bronx, NY 10467
Attn: Charles Pollak, M.D.

Sleep Disorders Center
Department of Psychiatry
SUNY at Stony Brook
Stony Brook, NY 11794
Attn: Merrill M. Mitler, Ph.D.

Sleep Disorders Center
Univ. of Cincinnati Hospital
Cincinnati, OH 45267
Attn: Milton Kramer, M.D.

Sleep Disorders Center
Mt. Sinai Hospital
University Circle
Cleveland, OH 44106
Attn: Herbert Weiss, M.D.

Sleep Disorders Center
Department of Psychiatry
Ohio State University
Columbus, OH 43210
Attn: Helmut Schmidt, M.D.

Sleep Disorders Center
Presbyterian Hospital
N.E. 13th at Lincoln Blvd.
Oklahoma City, OK 73104
Attn: William Orr, Ph.D.

Sleep Disorders Center
Western Psychiatric Institute
3811 O'Hara Street
Pittsburgh, PA 15261
Attn: David Kupfer, M.D.

Sleep Disorders Center
Department of Neurology
Crozer-Chester Med. Center
Upland – Chester, PA 19013
Attn: Calvin Stafford, M.D.

BMH Sleep Disorders Center
Baptist Memorial Hospital
Memphis, TN 38146
Attn: Helio Lemmi, M.D.

Sleep Disorders Center
Baylor College of Medicine
Houston, TX 77030
Attn: Ismet Karacan, M.D.

Sleep Disorders Center
Metropolitan Medical Center
1303 McCullough
San Antonio, TX 78212
Attn: J. Catesby Ware, Ph.D.

Developing centers

Sleep Disorders Center
Neurosciences – Box 190
University of Alabama
Birmingham, AL 35294
Attn: Vernon Pegram, Ph.D.

Sleep Laboratory
Department of Pulmonary Medicine
Univ. of Arkansas Med. Center
Little Rock, AR 72201
Attn: Edgar Lucas, Ph.D.

Sleep Disorders Center
Good Samaritan Hospital
1033 East McDowell Road
Phoenix, AZ 85006
Attn: Bernard E. Levine, M.D.

Sleep Disorders Center
Department of Neurology
UCLA School of Medicine
Los Angeles, CA 90024
Attn: Emery Zimmerman, M.D., Ph.D.

Sleep Disorders Center
The Griffin Hospital
130 Division Street
Derby, CN 06418
Attn: Robert Watson, Ph.D.

Sleep Disorders Center
National Jewish Hospital
3800 East Colfax Avenue
Denver, CO 80206
Attn: David Shucard, Ph.D.

Sleep Disorders Clinic
Boston Children's Hospital
300 Longwood Avenue
Boston, MA 02115
Attn: Richard Ferber, M.D.

Sleep Disorders Unit
Beth Israel Hospital
330 Brookline Avenue
Boston, MA 02215
Attn: Michael P. Biber, M.D.

Sleep Center
755 W. Big Beaver Rd.
Suite 2009
Troy, MI 48084
Attn: Harvey Halberstadt, M.D.

Sleep Laboratory
Division of Pulmonary Medicine
Mayo Clinic
Rochester, MN 55901
Attn: Phillip Westbrook, M.D.

Sleep Disorders Center
Med. Sciences Building
New Jersey Med. School
Newark, NJ 07103
Attn: James Minard, Ph.D.

Sleep Disorders Center
Rutgers Medical School
Box 101
Piscataway, NJ 08502
Attn: Leonide Goldstein, D.Sc.

Sleep Disorders Center
VA Medical Center
Irving Avenue
Syracuse, NY 13210
Attn: Antonio Culebras, M.D.

Sleep Disorders Center
Psychiatry Department
St. Luke's Hospital
Cleveland, OH 44118
Attn: Joel Steinberg, M.D.

Sleep Disorders Center
Shoal Creek Hospital
3501 Mills Avenue
Austin, TX 78731
Attn: J. Douglas Hudson, M.D.

Sleep Disorders Center
Utah Neurological Clinic
1999 N. Columbia Lane
Provo, UT 84601
Attn: John M. Andrews, M.D.

Canadian centers

Sleep Disorders Clinic
Hopital du Sacre-Coeur
5400 ouest, Boul. Gouin
Montreal, Qu., CANADA H4J 1C5
Attn: Jacques Montplaisir, M.D.

Sleep Disorders Clinic-Neurology
Ottawa General Hospital
43 Bruyere
Ottawa, CANADA K1N 5C8
Attn: Roger Broughton, M.D.

Sleep Disorders Center
Sunnybrook Medical Center
2075 Bayview Avenue
Toronto, CANADA
Attn: Mortimer Mamelak, M.D.

Sleep Disorders Clinic
Department of Psychiatry
Toronto Western Hospital
Toronto, CANADA M5T 2S8
Attn: Harvey Moldofsky, M.D.

Other centers

Department of Neurology
Charles University
Katerinska 30
12000 Prague 2, CZECHOSLOVAKIA
Attn: B. Roth, M.D.

Service: Sommeil-Reve
Hospital Neurologique
39, boulevard Pinel
69500 Bron – FRANCE
Attn: Professeur M. Jouvet

Laboratoire de Medicine Experimental
Instiue de Biologie
Boulevard Henri IV
34000 Montpellier, FRANCE
Attn: Dr. P. Passouant

Clinica delle Malattie
Mervose et Mentali
Universita di Bologna
Bologna, ITALIA
Attn: Dr. E. Lugaresi

Department of Neuropsychiatry
Osaka University Medical School
1–1–50 Fukushima
Osaka, JAPAN 533
Attn: Dr. Y. Hishikawa

Department of Neuropsychiatry
Kurume University School of Medicine
67 Asahi–machi
Kurume, JAPAN 830
Attn: Dr. Y. Nakazawa

Department of Psychiatry
Tokyo University School of Medicine
7–3–1 Hongo, Bunkyo-ku
Tokyo, JAPAN 113
Attn: Dr. Y. Honda

Sleep Disorders Center
First Moscow Medical Institute
Moscow, U.S.S.R.
Attn: Professor A. Vein

Your Sleep Diary Bedtime Log

Continue to Day 14 or Day 21

	Day 1	Day 2	Day 3	Day 4
Date:				
Sleepiness, on a scale of 1 to 10: 1 2 3 4 5 6 7 8 9 10 alert drowsy extremely tired				
Mood, on a scale of 1 to 10: 1 2 3 4 5 6 7 8 9 10 anxious tense relaxed				
Describe activities from dinner until bedtime.				
Presleep ritual: describe each step up to getting in bed.				
What was the actual time you got into bed?				
Describe activities before lights-out.				
Did you take a sleeping pill? If so, write down name and amount.				
Have you had any alcohol in the past four hours? If so, write down what and how much you drank.				
How much coffee have you had today? In the last six hours?				

Your Sleep Diary Bedtime Log, cont.

Continue to Day 14 or Day 21

	Day 1	Day 2	Day 3	Day 4
How many cigarettes have you smoked today? In the last six hours?				
What time did you eat dinner?				
What have you eaten since dinner?				
Have you used any drugs (prescription and nonprescription) today? List specific drugs and amount used.				
Have you had any physical problems or discomfort during the day? If so, describe.				
Have you had any unusually stressful experiences today? Have you felt particularly relaxed, uptight, sad, or elated?				
Did you exercise during the day? Indicate what you did and when.				
Sum up your thoughts and feelings about your day.				

Your Sleep Diary Wake-Up Log

Continue to Day 14 or Day 21

	Day 1	Day 2	Day 3	Day 4
Estimate the time you fell asleep last night.				
Did you wake up in the night? How often? How long did you stay awake each time?				
What did you do when you awakened in the night?				
What time did you wake up in the morning?				
Did you wake up before or after the alarm?				
What time did you get out of bed?				
Indicate how well you slept on a scale of 1 to 10: 1 2 3 4 5 6 7 8 9 10 very poorly very well				
Indicate your energy level on a scale of 1 to 10: 1 2 3 4 5 6 7 8 9 10 very tired groggy refreshed, energetic				
Estimate your total sleep time during the night.				

Your Sleep Diary Dinner-Time Log:

Continue to Day 14 or Day 21

	Day 1	Day 2	Day 3	Day 4
Were you extremely sleepy during the morning or during the afternoon?				
Did you take any naps? When? For how long?				
How much time did you sleep during the day?				
Estimate how much time you have slept in the past twenty-four hours.				
Describe your functioning (creativity, concentration, decision-making, and so on) in the morning and in the afternoon on a scale of 1 to 10: 1 2 3 4 5 6 7 8 9 10 inadequate adequate peak, outstanding				
Using the same scale, describe your feelings and ability to cope in the morning and in the afternoon.				
Describe your emotions during the day.				
Describe your physical state during the day.				

Glossary

Alpha Rhythm: Electrical activity of the brain during wakefulness. Most consistent and predominant during relaxation, particularly when visual stimulation is reduced. Frequency ranges from 8–13 Hz (cycles per second) and varies with age. Slower in children and older age groups, compared to young and middle-aged adults.

Arousal: Abrupt change from "deep" sleep (Stage 3 or 4) or from REM sleep to wakefulness. Awakening is considered full arousal.

Cataplexy: A sudden, dramatic loss of muscle tone, leading to muscle weakness, paralysis or collapse; usually triggered by an emotional outburst, such as laughter or anger. One of the characteristic symptoms of narcolepsy.

Circadian Rhythm: The daily fluctuation in physiological and behavioral functions over a period of about 24 hours.

"Deep" Sleep: Common term for Stages 3 and 4 of sleep.

Delta Rhythm: Electrical activity during the deep sleep of Stages 3 and 4.

Hypersomnia: Excessive or prolonged sleep, sometimes associated with difficulty in awakening or sleep drunkenness.

Hypnagogic Hallucinations: Vivid visual or auditory perceptions occurring before or after sleep. Characteristic of narcolepsy.

Insomnia: A general term for any difficulty in sleeping.

"Light" Sleep: Common term for Stage 1 and sometimes Stage 2 NREM sleep.

Myoclonus: Muscle contractions in the form of jerks or twitches.

Nightmare: A term that denotes a dream anxiety attack.

NREM Sleep: Stages 1, 2, 3 and 4 of sleep, which are characterized by an absence of rapid eye movements; also referred to as non-REM sleep.

Polysomnogram: Continuous, simultaneous recording of several physiological variables (primarily brain activity, eye movements and muscular activity) during sleep.

REM Sleep: The stage of sleep characterized by rapid eye movements, intense brain activity, suppressed muscle activity and vivid dreams.

REM Latency: The period of time from sleep onset to the first REM period.

REM Rebound: A lengthening and increase in REM periods following REM deprivation.

Sleep Onset: The transition from waking to sleep; the time from lights-out to sleep.

Sleep Pattern: An individual's 24-hour schedule for waking and resting.

Stage 1 Sleep: A stage of NREM sleep that serves as the transition from waking to sleep.

Stage 2 Sleep: A stage of NREM sleep that accounts for 45 to 55 percent of the total sleep time of adults; sometimes described as a "filler" state.

Stage 3 Sleep: A stage of NREM sleep that is characterized by the appearance of slow delta brain waves and produces deep rest; appears in the first third of the night.

Stage 4 Sleep: A stage of NREM sleep characterized by delta brain waves; the deepest, most profound sleep state.

Slow Wave Sleep: A term used to describe Stages 3 and 4 of NREM sleep.

Tumescence (penile): Hardening and expansion of the penis. If it occurs during sleep, referred to as nocturnal penile tumescence.

Glossary definitions are adapted from the diagnostic classification of the Association of Sleep Disorders Centers and the Association for the Psychophysiological Study of Sleep.

Bibliography

Part I: The facts of sleep

General background

Cartwright, R. *A Primer of Sleep and Dreaming.* Reading, Mass.: Addison-Wesley, 1978.

Dement, W.C. and Mitler, M.M. "An Overview of Sleep Research: Past, Present and Future." In *American Handbook of Psychiatry,* edited by D. Hamburg and K. Brodie. Vol. 6. New York: Basic Books, 1976.

Dement, William C. *Some Must Watch While Some Must Sleep.* San Francisco: San Francisco Book Company, 1976.

Drucker-Colin, R., Shkurovich, M. and Sterman M. (eds.). *The Functions of Sleep.* New York: Academic Press, 1979.

Foulkes, David. *The Psychology of Sleep.* New York: Charles Scribner's Sons, 1966.

Hobson, J. Allan. *The Ethology of Sleep.* Nutley, N.J.: Hoffman-La Roche, 1979.

Kleitman, Nathaniel. *Sleep and Wakefulness.* Chicago, University of Chicago Press, 1963.

Medical Times, Vol. 107, No. 6. June, 1979. (Issue devoted to sleep problems.)

Psychiatric Annals, Vol. 9, Nos. 7 and 8, July and August, 1979. (Both issues devoted to sleep disorders.)

Segal, Julius and Luce, Gay Gaer. *Sleep.* New York: Coward-McCann, 1966.

Webb, Wilse B. *Sleep: The Gentle Tyrant.* New York: Prentice-Hall, 1975.

Williams, R.L. et al. *Electroencephalography (EEG) of Human Sleep: Clinical Applications.* New York: John Wiley, 1974.

Circadian rhythms

Halberg, F. "Implications of Biological Rhythms for Clinical Practice." *Hospital Practice* 12: 139–149, January 1977.

Leff, D.N. "Chronobiologists Tell Clinicians: Think Circadian." *Medical World News* 44–53, July 23, 1979.

Luce, Gay Gaer. *Body Time.* New York: Pantheon Books, 1971.

Richter, C.P. *Biological Clocks in Medicine and Psychiatry.* Springfield, Ill.: C.C. Thomas, 1966.

Scheving, L.E. "Chronobiology and Its Relationship to Developing a Knowledge Base for Regulating Decisions about Health and Prevention." *Chronobiologia* 6, Jan–March 1979.

Dreams

Cartwright, R.D. et al. "Focusing on Dreams: A Preparatory Program for Psychotherapy." *Archives of General Psychiatry* 37: 275–277, 1980.

———. "Happy Endings for our Dreams." *Psychology Today* 12: 66–77, December 1978.

———. *Nightlife: Explorations in Dreaming.* New Jersey: Prentice-Hall, 1977.

———. "The Nature and Function of Repetitive Dreams: A Survey and Speculations." *Psychiatry* 42: 131, May 1979.

Delaney, Gayle. *Living Your Dreams.* New York: Harper and Row, 1979.

Diamond, Edwin. *The Science of Dreams.* New York: Doubleday, 1962.

Foulkes, D. "Dreams of Innocence." *Psychology Today* 12: 78–88, December, 1978.

Garfield, Patricia. *Creative Dreaming.* New York: Simon & Schuster, 1974.

Hobson, J.A. and McCarley, R.W. "The Brain as a Dream State Generator: An Activation-Synthesis Hypothesis of the Dream Process." *American Journal of Psychiatry* 134: 1335–1348, December, 1977.

———. "The Neurobiological Origins of Psychoanalytical Dream Theory." *American Journal of Psychiatry* 134: 1211–21, November, 1977.

Kramer, M. (ed.). *Dream Psychology and the New Biology of Dreaming.* Springfield, Ill.: C.C. Thomas, 1969.

McCarley, R.W. "Where Dreams Come From: A New Theory." *Psychology Today* 12: 54–65, December, 1978.

Sleeping brain

Arkin, A.M., Antrobus, J.S. and Ellman, S.J. (eds.). *The Mind in Sleep: Psychology and Psychophysiology.* Hillsdale, N.J.: Lawrence Erlbaum Associates, 1978.

Budzynski, T. "Tuning In on the Twilight Zone." *Psychology Today,* August 1977, pp. 39–44.

Cartwright, R. "Sleep Fantasy in Normal and Schizophrenic Patients." *Journal of Abnormal Psychology* 80: 275–279, 1972.

Clemes, S.R. and Dement, W.C. "Effect of REM Sleep Deprivation on Psychological Functioning." *Journal of Nervous and Mental Disease* 144: 485–91, 1967.

Corfman, E. *Depression, Manic-Depressive Illness and Biological Rhythms.* Bethesda, Md.: National Institute of Mental Health, 1979.

Hawkins, D. "Sleep and Depression." *Psychiatric Annals* 9: 13–28, August, 1979.

Hockey, G.R.J. "Forgetting as a Function of Sleep and Different Times of Day." *Quarterly Journal of Experimental Psychology* 24: 386–393, 1972.

Hoddes, Eric. "Does Sleep Help You Study"? *Psychology Today,* June 1977, p. 69.

Mendels, J. and Hawkins, D. "Sleep and Depression." *Archives of General Psychiatry* 344–354, 1967.

Reich, L. et al. "Sleep Disturbance in Schizophrenia." *Archives of General Psychiatry.* 32: 51–55, 1975.

Wehr, T.A. et al. "Phase Advance of the Circadian Sleep-Wake Cycle as an Antidepressant." *Science* 206: 0, November 9, 1979.

Vogel, G. and Traub, A. "REM Deprivation: The Effect on Schizophrenic Patients." *Archives of General Psychiatry* 18: 287–329, 1968.

Vogel, G.W. et al. "Improvement of Depression by REM Sleep Deprivation." *Archives of General Psychiatry* 37: 247–253, March 1980.

Zarcone, V. "Sleep and Schizophrenia." *Psychiatric Annals* 9: 29–40, August, 1979.

Part II: Sleep sense

General background

Bergamasco, B. et al. "Human Sleep Modifications Induced by Urban Traffic Noise." *Acta Otolaryn. Supplement* 339: 33–36, 1976.

Dullea G. "Doing Business in the Bedroom." *New York Times,* August 6, 1980.

Dunkell, Samuel. *Sleep Positions: The Night Language of the Body.* NAL 1978.

Friedman, J. et al. "Changes in Sleep Patterning with Reduction of Night Aircraft Noise at Los Angeles International Airport." *Sleep Research* 6: 127, 1977.

Gallup Pool of Sleeping Habits. Nutley, N.J.: Hoffman-La Roche, 1980.

Hartmann, E. et al. "Psychological Differences between Long and Short Sleepers." *Archives of General Psychiatry* 26: 463–468, May 1972.

Hinds, M.D. "For the Sleep That Refreshes." *New York Times,* February 6, 1980.

Karacan, I. et al. "Erection Cycle During Sleep in Relation to Dream Anxiety." *Archives of General Psychiatry* 15: 183–189, 1966.

Kaya, N. et al. Nocturnal Penile Tumescence and its Role in Impotence." *Psychiatric Annals* 9: 63–68, August 1979.

Kilich B. "Bedroom with a Double Life." *San Francisco Chronicle,* August 6, 1980.

Kleiman, C. "New Sleep Research: Why Your Dream Life Is Different from His." *Ms.,* August 1979, p. 28–30.

Parlee, M.B. "The Temperatures of a Marriage." *Psychology Today,* June 1979, p. 29.

Segal, J. "How Do You Feel After Sex—Sleepy or Exhilarated"? *Glamour,* May 1978, pp. 78, 86.

Silva, R. "Drifting and Dreaming." *Off-Duty, West.* September, 1979.

Switzer, E. and Langmyhr, G. "Your Sex Life and How It Affects the Way You Sleep." *Vogue,* August 1973, pp. 120–121, 148.

Tracy, R. "Environmental Noise Affects the Quality of Sleep." Better Sleep Council. December 31, 1979.

———. "Majority Nap to Replace Lost Sleep." Better Sleep Council. October 22, 1979.

———. "Phantom Noises Can Damage the Quality of Your Sleep." Better Sleep Council, September 11, 1978.

———. "Today's Woman: Even Her Dreams Are Changing." Better Sleep Council, April 10, 1978.

———. "Whatever Happened to the Bedroom"? Better Sleep Council, November 12, 1979.

Webb, W.B. "Sleep and Naps." *Speculations in Science and Technology* 1:3; 3–318, 1978.

Part II: Alternative therapies

Alternative therapies

Bootzin, R.R. and Nicassio, P. "Behavioral Treatments for Insomnia." In *Progress in Behavior Modification,* edited by M. Herson et al. New York: Academic Press, 1978.

Bootzin, R.R. "Effects of Self-Control Procedures for Insomnia." In *Behavioral Self-Management Strategies, Techniques and Outcomes,* edited by R.B. Stuart. New York: Bruner-Mazel, 1977.

Coates, Thomas J. and Thoresen, Carl E. *How to Sleep Better.* Englewood Cliffs, N.J.: Prentice-Hall, 1977.

———. "Treating Arousals during Sleep Using Behavioral Self-Management." *Journal of Consulting and Clinical Psychology,* in press.

Goldberg, Philip and Kaufman, Daniel. *Natural Sleep.* Emmaus, Pa.: Rodale Press, 1978.

Hauri, P. "Behavioral Treatment of Insomnia." *Medical Times* 107: 36–47, 1979.

Hauri, P. and Cohen, S. "The Treatment of Insomnia with Biofeedback: Final Report of Study I." *Sleep Research* 6: 136, 1977.

Knapp, T.J. et al. "Behavior Therapy for Insomnia: A Review and Critique." *Behavior Therapy* 7: 614–625, 1976.

Regestein, Q.R. "Practical Ways to Manage Chronic Insomnia." *Medical Times* 107: 19–23, June 1979.

Segal, Julius and Luce, Gay Gaer. *Insomnia: The Guide for Troubled Sleepers.* New York: Doubleday, 1969.

Sleeping pills

Balter, M.D. and Bauer, M.L. "Patterns of Prescribing and Use of Hypnotic Drugs in the United States." In *Sleep Disturbances and Hypnotic Drug Dependence,* edited by A.D. Clif. Amsterdam: Excerpta Medica, 1975.

Church, M.W. and Johnson, L.C. "Mood and Performance of Poor Sleepers during Repeated Use of Flurazepam." *Psychopharmacology* 61: 309–316, 1979.

Dement W. and Zarcone V. "Pharmacological Treatment of Sleep Disorders." In *Psycho-Pharmacology from Therapy to Practice,* edited by J.D. Barchas and R.D. Ciarenello. New York: Oxford University Press, 1977.

"Drugs for Human Use: Over-the-Counter Daytime Sedatives." *Federal Register,* Vol. 44, No. 122, June 22, 1979.

Gillin, J.C. et al. "Flurazepam and Insomnia." *Science* 205: 954–955, September 7, 1979.

Hartmann, Ernest. *The Sleeping Pill.* New Haven: Yale University Press, 1978.

Harvey, S.C. "Hypnotics and Sedatives, The Barbiturates." In *Pharmacological Basis of Therapeutics* (edited by L. Goodman and A. Gillman.) New York: MacMillan, 1975.

Hauri, P. "Aspirin and Insomnia." Sleep Research 7, 1978.

Kales J. et al. "Are OTC Sleep Medications Effective"? *Current Therapeutic Research* 13, March 31, 1973.

Kripke, D.F. et al. "Short and Long Sleep and Sleeping Pills." *Archives of General Psychiatry* 36: 103–116, January 1979.

Kripke, D.F. et al. "Sleep Duration, Insomnia and Sleeping Pill Use." *Archives of General Psychiatry* 36: 103–116, 1979.

Miller, R.R. "A Guide to the Use of Hypnotic Drugs." *Medical Times* 107: 28–35, June 1979.

"Over-the-Counter Nighttime Sleep Aids and Stimulating Products: Tentative Final Orders." *Federal Register.* June 13, 1978.

Sedative Hypnotic Drugs: Risks and Benefits. National Institute on Drug Abuse, 1977.

Sleeping Pills, Insomnia and Medical Practice. Report of a Study by a Committee of the Institute of Medicine, National Academy of Sciences, Washington, D.C., 1979.

Solomon, F. et al. "Special Report: Sleeping Pills, Insomnia and Medical Practice." *New England Journal of Medicine* 300: 803, 1979.

Williams, R. and Karacan, I. *Pharmacology of Sleep.* New York: John Wiley, 1976.

Part III: Making it through the night

General background on sleep disorders

Bixler, E.O. et al. "Incidence of Sleep Disorders in Medical Practice: A Physician Survey." *Sleep Research* 5: 160, 1976.

Dement, W.C. "Normal Sleep and Sleep Disorders." In *Psychiatry in General Medical Practice,* edited by G. Usdin and J. Lewis. New York: McGraw-Hill, 1979.

Dement, William and Guilleminault, Christian (eds.). *Sleep.* Vol. II, No. 1. New York: Raven Press, 1980.

Hauri, Peter. *The Sleep Disorders.* Kalamazoo, Mich.: Upjohn, 1977.

Mendelson, Wallace, Gillin, J. Christian and Wyatt, Richard (eds.). *Human Sleep and its Disorders.* New York: Plenum Press, 1977.

Monroe, L.J. "Psychological and Physiological Differences between Good and Poor Sleepers." *Journal of Abnormal Psychology* 72: 255–264, 1967.

Regestein, Q.R. "Chronic Insomnia Provikes More Prescriptions than Diagnoses." *Journal of the American Medical Association* 237: 1569.

―――. "Treating Insomnia: A Practical Guide for Managing Chronic Sleeplessness, circa 1975." *Comprehensive Psychiatry* 17: 517–526, 1976.

Usdin, G. and Hawkins, D. *The Office Guide to Sleep Disorders.* New York: KPR Infor/Media, 1980.

Ware, J.C. "The Symptom of Insomnia: Causes and Cures." *Psychiatric Annals* 9: 353–365, 1979.

Williams, Robert and Karacan, Ismet (eds.). *Sleep Disorders: Diagnosis and Treatment.* New York: John Wiley, 1978.

Problems falling asleep

Ekbom, K.A. "Restless Legs Syndrome." *Neurology* 10: 868–873, 1960.

Frankel, B.L. et al. "Restless Legs Syndrome." *Journal of the American Medical Association* 230: 1302–1303, December 2, 1974.

Goldstein A. and Kaizer Z. "Psychotropic Effects of Caffeine in Man." *Clinical Pharmacology and Therapeutics* 10: 477–488.

Hartse, K.M. et al. "Rebound Insomnia." *Science* 208: 423, April 25, 1980.

Hirsch, B. "Smoke Signals." *Psychology Today,* September 1980, p. 23.

Kales, A. et al. "Rebound Insomnia." *Journal of the American Medical Association* 241: 1692–1695, April 20, 1979.

Problems staying asleep

Baird, W.P. "Sleep Apnea: A Non-Medical Presentation." Palo Alto, Ca.: American Narcolepsy Association, 1977.

Brody, J.E. "The Search for a Cure for Snoring." *New York Times*, May 21, 1980.

Broughton, R.J. "The Incubus Attack." *International Psychiatric Clinics* 7: 188–192, 1970.

———. "Sleep Disorders: Disorders of Arousal"? *Science* 159: 1070–1078, 1968.

Fisher, C. et al. "A Psychophysiological Study of Nightmares and Night Terrors." *Archives of General Psychiatry* 28: 252–259, 1973.

Glaros, A.G. and Rao, S.M. "Bruxism: A Critical Review." *Psychological Bulletin* 84: 767–781, 1977.

Greenberg, R. "Dream Interruption Insomnia." *Journal of Nervous and Mental Disease* 144: 18–21, 1967.

Guilleminault, C. "The Sleep Apnea Syndrome." *Medical Times*, June, 1979, pp. 59–67.

Guilleminault, C. and Dement, W. (eds.). *Sleep Apnea Syndromes*. New York: Allen R. Liss, 1978.

Harris, I.D. "The Dream of the Object Endangered." *Psychiatry* 20: 151–161, 1957.

———. "Characterological Significance of the Typical Anxiety Dreams." *Psychiatry* 14: 279–294, 1951.

———. "Observations Concerning Typical Anxiety Dreams." *Psychiatry* 11: 301–309, 1948.

———. "Typical Anxiety Dreams and Object Relations." *International Journal of Psychoanalysis* 41: 604–611, 1960.

Hartmann, E. "Alcohol and Bruxism." *New England Journal of Medicine* 301: 333–334, 1979.

Hartmann, E. et al. "The Personality of the Nightmare Sufferer: Relationship to Schizophrenia." *Proceedings*, 18th Annual Meeting of the Association for the Psychophysiological Study of Sleep, Palo Alto, CA., 1978.

Hersen, M. "Personality Characteristics of Nightmare Sufferers." *Journal of Nervous and Mental Disease* 153: 27–31, 1971.

Kales, A. et al. "Clinical and Psychological Characteristics of Patients with Night Terrors." *Sleep Research* 6: 148, 1977.

———. "Clinical Characteristics of Patients with Night Terrors: Further Studies." *Proceedings*, 18th Annual Meeting of the Association for the Psychophysiological Study of Sleep. Palo Alto, Ca., 1978.

———. "Sleepwalking and Night Terrors Related to Febrile Illness." *American Journal of Psychiatry* 136: 1214–1215, September 1979.

Kramer, M. "Dream Disturbances." *Psychiatric Annals* 9: 50–68, July 1979.

Mitler, M.M. et al. "Sleeplessness, Sleep Attacks and Things That Go Wrong in the Night." *Psychology Today*, December 1975, p. 46.

Reding, G. et al. "Sleep Patterns of Tooth-grinding." *Science* 145: 725–726, 1964.

Problems of waking

Kupfer, D.J. "Sleep Disorders in Depression." In *Depression and Antidepressants,* edited by E. Friedman et al. New York: Raven Press, in press.

Pokorny, A.D. "Sleep Disturbances, Alcohol and Alcoholism: A Review." In *Sleep Disorders: Diagnosis and Treatment,* edited by R.L. Williams and I. Karacan. New York: John Wiley, pp. 233–260.

Problems of excessive daytime sleepiness

Baird, W.P. "Narcolepsy." Palo Alto, Ca.: American Narcolepsy Association, 1977.

Dement, W. et al. "Narcolepsy: A Major Cause of Excessive Sleepiness." *Consultant* 17: 25–28, 1977.

Dement, W.C. "Narolepsy: Not As Rare As We Believed." *Medical Times,* June 1979, pp. 51–55.

Guilleminault C. et al. (eds.). *Narcolepsy.* New York: Spectrum, 1976.

Karacan, I. et al. "The Narcoleptic Syndrome." *Psychiatric Annals* 9: 69–76, July 1979.

Orr, W.C. et al. "When to Suspect Sleep Apnea: The 'Pickwickian Syndrome.'" *Medical Times,* July 1978.

Simmons, F.B. et al. "Surgical Management of Airway Obstructions During Sleep." *The Laryngoscope* 87: 326–338, March, 1977.

Zarcone, V. "Narcolepsy." *New England Journal of Medicine* 288: 1156–1163, May 31, 1973.

Occasional sleep problems

Goldberg, V. "What Can We Do About Jet Lag"? *Psychology Today,* August, 1977, p. 69–72.

Kripke, D.F. et al. "Sleep of Night Workers." *Psychophysiology* 7: 377–384, 1971.

Williams, R.L. *Sleep Disturbances in Various Medical and Surgical Conditions.* In

Williams, R.L. "Sleep Disturbances in Various Medical and Surgical Conditions." In *Sleep Disorders: Diagnosis and Treatment,* edited by R.L. Williams and I. Karacan. New York: John Wiley, 1977.

Children's sleep problems

Anders, T. and Weinstein, P. "Sleep and Its Disorders in Infants and Children." *Pediatrics* 50: 312, 1972.

Doleys, D.M. "Behavioral Treatments for Nocturnal Enuresis in Children. A Review of Recent Literature." *Psychological Bulletin* 84: 30–58, 1977.

Facts about Sudden Infant Death Syndrome. National Institute of Child Health and Human Development, Bethesda, Md., 1972.

Ferber, K. and Rivinus, T. "Practical Approaches to Sleep Disorders of Childhood." *Medical Times,* June 1979, pp. 72–80.

Guilleminault, C. and Anders, T. "Sleep Disorders in Children." *Advances in Pediatrics* 22: 151–174, 1976.

Lennert, J.B. and Moward, J.J. "Enuresis: Evaluation of a Perplexing Symptom." *Urology* XIII, 27–29, January 1979.

Lipsett, L. "Conditioning the Rage to Live." *Psychology Today,* February 1980, p. 124.

Moore, T. and Ucko, L.E. "Night Waking in Early Infancy." *Archives of Disease of Children* 32: 333–342, 1957.

Sleep problems of the elderly

Feinberg, I. "Functional Implications of Changes in Sleep Physiology with Age." In *Neurobiology of Aging,* edited by R.D. Terry. New York: Raven Press, 1976.

Prinz, P. "Sleep Patterns in the Healthy Aged: Relationship with Intellectual Function." *Journal of Gerontology* 32: 1979–186, 1977.

Prinz, P. and Raskin, M. "Aging and Sleep Disorders." In *Sleep Disorders: Diagnosis and Treatment,* edited by R. Williams and I. Karacan. New York: John Wiley, 1978.

Regestein, Q. "Sleep and Insomnia in the Elderly." *Journal of Geriatric Psychiatry,* in press.

Index

Adapin (doxepin), 145

Adolescence: depression, 214, 235; dreams in, 270; Kleine-Levin Syndrome, 85, 233, menstrual periods, 32, 86, 248; sleep needs, 214, 235, 257; sleep paralysis, 217; "wet" dreams, 88

Age: and irregular hours, 243; and quality of sleep, 276; and REM latency, 60; and sleep needs, 98, 276–278; and sleep patterns, 31, 60, 275–276; and sleeping problems, 10, 227

Aged. *See* Elderly

Aging, 21, 32, 55, 276–277

Alcohol: after dinner, 171; and dreams, 37, 45, 58, 220; and NREM-REM cycles, 37; and other drugs, 38, 132, 133, 135, 136, 138, 140; overindulgence in, 99–100, 104, 219–220, 232; withdrawal from, 37

American Association for the Psychophysiological Study of Sleep, 13

American Narcolepsy Association (ANA), 226

Amnesia, 235

Amphetamines, 183, 226, 231

Amytol (amobarbitol), 135–137

Angina, 246

Animals: bed area, 67; biological hour, 21; dreams of, 49, 50, 59; sex and sleep, 90, 91; sleep cycles of, 15–16; time cues for, 17

Anticonvulsant drugs, 200

Antidepressant drugs, 145, 205, 208, 215–216, 226

Antihistamines, 134, 144–145, 230, 232; nonprescription, 147, 150–151; overdose, 147

Antipsychotic drugs, 145

Anxiety, 171–174

Apnea, 225, 245; causes of, 193–194, 228–229; in children, 194, 261, 271–272; death risk in, 191, 195, 227; diagnosis and treatment of, 194–195, 229–230, 290; drugs and, 132, 195, 281; in the elderly, 35, 227, 281; in infants, 194; sexual differences in, 85, 227. *See also* Central sleep apnea; Obstructive sleep apnea

Association of Sleep Disorders Centers (ASDC), 12–13

Asthma, 35, 246

Aspirin, 18, 146, 147–148

Athletes, 38–39, 43

Attention span, 21–22

Attributional therapy, 126–127

Autogenic training, 116

Backache, 72

Barbituates, 135–137. *See also* Sleeping pills

Bed board, 72

Bedroom: compatibility in, 93; contemporary, 69–70, 75; darkness in, 80; evolution of, 67–69; mood, 75–76; other uses for, 70; personality reflection of, 76–77; temperature of, 76, 77–78, 80–81

Beds: ancient, 68; how to buy, 73-74; size of, 71, 94; water, 73. *See also* Mattresses

Bed-wetting (enuresis), 207, 228; causes of, 204–205; in children, 204–205, 264–266, 271, 273; heredity and, 30–31; sexual differences in, 85; treatment of, 205, 265–266

Benadryl (dephenhydramine), 145

Benedek, Therese, 87

Benzodiazepines, 137–139

Bettelheim, Bruno, 268–269

Biofeedback, 122–124, 197

Biological rhythms: and administration of medication, 18–20; age changes, 277–278; and delayed sleep onset, 179–180; energy levels and attention span, 21, 25; irregular, 180–182; and learning, 22. *See also* Sleep/wake cycles

Biorhythms, 17–18

Blankets, 76, 77, 93

Blind people, 17, 58

Blood pressure, 246

Body movements, rhythmic, 197–199. *See also* Children; Infants; Head-banging; Leg jerks; Restless leg syndrome; Rocking

Body temperature: and performance, 22, 24; in pregnancy, 250; rhythmic changes in, 16, 17; in sleep, 7, 77; and sleep disorders, 24, 179

Bootzin, Richard, 120, 176

Brain: age and, 55, 277; and body temperature changes, 22; chemical changes in, 17; and dreams, 49–50; dysfunction, 233; and jet lag, 26-27; monitoring, 12; sensory images in, 57–59; in sleep, 5, 6, 53–63, 224; workings of, 53–55

Breathing: normal patterns of, 6–7; for relaxation, 118. *See also* Apnea; Snoring

Brevital (methohexital), 136

Bromides, 146

Bruxism. *See* Teeth grinding

Butisol (butobarbital), 136

Butler, Robert, 282

Caffeine, 36, 104, 169, 170–171, 178, 182–185, 225, 231

Cancer patients, 19, 20

Cardiac arrhythmia, 194, 247, 271

Carskadon, Mary, 11, 110